Dear Joh

more courage,
more curiosity,
more compassion!

Tamara

# #WHATIS

# #WHATIS
## MINDFULNESS?

## DR TAMARA RUSSELL

This edition first published in the UK and USA 2017 by
Watkins, an imprint of Watkins Media Limited
19 Cecil Court
London WC2N 4EZ

enquiries@watkinspublishing.com

1 3 5 7 9 10 8 6 4 2

Designed and typeset by Manisha Patel

Printed and bound in Germany

A CIP record for this book is available from the British Library

ISBN: 978-1-78678-015-7


www.watkinspublishing.com

# CONTENTS

# Why read this book?

My aim in writing this book is to provide you with a friendly, accessible guide to mindfulness – such a popular term these days, yet one that is rarely fully understood. I would like to give you a broad understanding of the topic, as well as clear up some common confusions. With more insight into the meaning, mechanisms and origins of mindfulness, I believe it's possible for everyone to find a way to weave mindfulness into their daily lives. I'm passionate about the brain and keen to share the exciting neuroscientific research that's helping us understand why mindfulness really can 'work'. As we all know, we need clear and calm thinking to meet the challenges our world is facing. Mindfulness is one route to ensuring we proceed with this consideration and clarity rather than knee-jerk reactions. In a more mindful world there is room for us all to thrive. I hope this book will inspire you to consider where in your world there is an opportunity to act with more care and attention, and in line with your deepest and most heartfelt intentions.

## 20 reasons to start reading!

1  Explore the meaning and concept of mindfulness
2  Differentiate between mindfulness and 'ordinary' awareness
3  Recognize that you already have mindfulness within you
4  Discover how mindful living benefits both body and mind
5  Understand the key brain networks you are using and
   developing when you practise mindfulness

6 Become familiar with different types of attention and how we can fine-tune our attentional capabilities

7 Get better acquainted with your wandering mind, and harness its power in line with your intentions

8 Learn how to learn in the most efficient ways

9 Understand the benefits of engaging with life's challenges in a less reactive, more considered way

10 Improve your self-knowledge and awareness of your own personal habits of mind

11 Feel confident you can make any activity mindful

12 Learn how developing awareness is in our genes

13 Hear the story of how many human civilizations have explored and developed awareness

14 Learn how modern-day mindfulness has grown into the globe-spanning phenomenon it is today

15 Learn how to prepare for mindfulness training, making your efforts most efficient

16 Discover how to be mindful in mindless environments

17 Reflect on your own personal learning style and how this will interact with attempts to unveil your innate mindfulness

18 Explore three key mindfulness practices in depth

19 Challenge yourself to embed mindfulness in everyday activities and interactions

20 Embrace the joy and pain of the human condition to continually learn and grow

From the list on the previous pages, you can see that I'm keen for you to explore this topic from all angles, so you really know what you are getting into if you decide that mindfulness is for you. Being prepared will speed your journey and make it more fun. You may explore lightly or want to go deep. You are at your own starting point and I hope that this book will give you all you need to know to begin your explorations.

## Key features of this book

In the Introduction that follows, I provide the context for this book and my work and my motivations for writing it. Chapter 1 explores the concept and the language of mindfulness, with Chapter 2 then elaborating on the brain activity that supports the special type of awareness we call mindfulness. Chapter 3 explores the origins of the practice, and our enduring fascination with expanding awareness, which continues to this day. Chapter 4 provides practical advice to help you consider the best way to approach mindfulness as an individual, and Chapter 5 provides practical exercises to help you get going. These are surprisingly simple with big impact when you engage with them in an informed way, knowing and understanding what your brain is doing. Finally, Chapter 6 considers what happens with continued, dedicated practice and whether it might be possible to create more mindful communities, and, ultimately, a more mindful world.

This book has a number of features to make mindfulness as accessible as possible for you. These include:

- A Q & A approach that, chapter by chapter, explores the questions that are often asked about mindfulness.
- 'Focus On' boxes that invite you to go deeper into a practice or topic and think about how it applies in your life.
- 'Try It' boxes that suggest practical exercises you can try right now to explore a learning/teaching point.
- At the end of the book, a 'What Next' section and further reading list suggest how to continue your investigations. This book is a first dip into the topic; if you really want to dive in, there are many more fascinating things to discover.

## KEY ABBREVIATIONS

The following abbreviations are used in the book for key terms (the terms themselves will be explained on first mention):

**MBSR** – Mindfulness-Based Stress Reduction
**MBCT** – Mindfulness-Based Cognitive Therapy
**DMN** – Default Mode Network

# INTRODUCTION

## Why this subject?

We are often overwhelmed in the media with articles and stories about mindfulness: how it can help with relationships, at work, in sports, with the management of emotions and the development of emotional intelligence. The list goes on! But how can it be that *one thing* can have an impact across so many areas of our life and society? How is it that mindfulness – in the many and various formats that we find it – can seem to have such a dramatic influence on people's lives? And as well as those who point to mindfulness as a panacea for what ails modern society, there are also plenty of sceptics. It is a fascinating and important subject, but what is the reality?

I have seen mindfulness, which is, at its core, a mind-training tool, benefit a wide range of people – from those who want to become more productive at work, to those who are seeking answers to larger, spiritual questions and those who just want more ease and gentleness in their life. However, there is huge variation in the way that it is and can be taught.

As this mental training technique has migrated from its beginnings in the monasteries to the mainstream, it has been adapted, reshaped and repositioned. While adaptations are to be encouraged, some of this reshaping has led to frustration and disappointment, as people are often left not really understanding how to do it or what to expect. At the heart of the ongoing debates we find a number of common misunderstandings about mindfulness. These misconceptions have proliferated as mindfulness has spread like wildfire through society.

Unrealistic expectations are one of the most common pitfalls. Some people believe they can achieve the full benefits of mindfulness if they spend just five minutes a day using an app on their morning commute. Although they *are* engaging in mindfulness training, it's important to make clear that this level of practice will not achieve the same results as, say, practising a body scan exercise almost every day for 45 minutes over 8 weeks (as in a standardized mindfulness training programme). And neither of these is likely to come close to what is attained by a lifelong practice and commitment to specific practices, in a specific order (as in the Buddhist training path). Yet, they are all ways of practising mindfulness.

Trying to find clarity even around the definition of 'mindfulness' in the secular domain has been problematic. Is it a state of mind, a training method or simply a way of being or doing? This book will define and discuss the key principles of mindfulness so you can gain a better understanding of it, explore how it can benefit your life and clarify what you want to achieve, how you plan to do it and what the likely rewards will be for your efforts.

Understanding the basics of the underlying theory and neuroscientific research behind mindfulness will help explain the how and why of certain practices, and help you think clearly about your intentions, expectations and associated effort and motivation if you take up mindfulness practice. As such, a simplified model for mindfulness will be presented that captures the key neuroscientific features of a focused attention process. Common confusions will be cleared up as we work our way through this, which will help you to refine your attempts at (or your existing) mindfulness practice and allow you to make more out of the time you are spending doing mindfulness.

I hope that the framework presented will also encourage those who are happy just to dip their toe into mindfulness. In particular, there are many in teaching or leadership roles who wish to take advantage of adding a little mindfulness to their work. Any activity can be done mindfully, and this book will be a helpful guide to any teachers and innovators who wish to try something new, but do so on the basis of solid brain science and cognitive theory.

In our time-poor society, it is helpful to act as efficiently as possible, and this book will allow your mindfulness journey to be more productive and help you be more confident that you are spending your time wisely.

## Why me?

I've come to my current understanding of mindfulness and the way it is taught through multiple routes. As a neuroscientist and clinical psychologist, trained at UCL and King's College London, I've been able to dive deep into the Western research that shows how and why mindfulness training is such a powerful tool in helping us live the life we want to lead. My personal training in kung fu and tai chi over almost 20 years has allowed me to sample the Eastern traditions, drawing out key mindfulness ideas and methods from this approach, too.

I am passionate about sharing this knowledge and have spent the last ten years talking to as many people as possible about mindfulness, its core features and training principles, and testing innovations to widen its scope and allow more people to connect to its potential.

I have visited hospitals, arts centres, festivals, conferences, and have even taught mindfulness at the top of London's Tower Bridge. Through this process, I have found out what lies at the heart of the practices, and the common barriers faced by us all in this modern life. I have seen directly that people do have it within them to use mindfulness to transform when given the right tools and support. I want to help facilitate this change in a way that's helpful and gives people the tools and choices to enable them to find their own path.

## Why now?

In recent years there has been an explosion of interest in mindfulness. It is now offered everywhere from healthcare settings and universities to large corporations, prisons and schools. Self-help books, online courses, apps and webinars all promise improved relationships and brains that work faster and more effectively. There is a huge amount of energy and positivity behind this surge in popularity, yet this rapid expansion may also have a cost. People who thought it would be a quick fix are becoming discouraged and all too quickly decide that it doesn't work for them.

As you read this book, it will become clear why mindfulness training is simple yet not easy. In part, this is because we live in a society that is fundamentally un-mindful. There is an overload of technology, we have shortened attention spans, high expectations, want instant gratification, and are not accustomed to being patient, quiet and still. We are also seeking to change neural networks that support the mental habits we wish to transform. This takes time and repetition. Change will not happen overnight, and to grasp this principle but also see that it *is* possible is the aim of this book.

We can regain real control, begin to reverse some of the unhelpful habits we have created, and wake up to what is possible in this life – all through mindfulness. At its core, mindfulness is being fully aware of what you are doing as you are doing it. When we develop this kind of deep awareness we see the impact of our current habitual ways of engaging with the world, technology and each other. With a non-judgemental curiosity and a commitment to learning and growing, we can begin to experiment with changing our habits. Those with the courage to persevere will notice that although it takes effort, it is worth it – relationships deepen, creativity emerges, and we better connect with the world and all the small moments that really make our life meaningful.

Today, people are asking bigger questions about what it really means to live in a mentally and physically healthy way, and what we really value. Now is also an amazing time when Eastern and Western models of health (and mind) are starting to merge. The mindfulness model described in this book represents a blending of the best of both of these worlds for the benefit of all.

As a scientist working at this time, I know we have an incredible opportunity to deepen our knowledge of the brain and mind. With this knowledge, it is possible for those interested in mindfulness to progress in ways that were previously just not feasible. So, now is the time, and this book holds the key. The journey is yours and here are the tools. The only question is... how far do you want to go?

# CHAPTER 1
What is mindfulness and
what are its benefits?

Mindfulness is, at its core, the ability to be fully aware of what you are doing, as you are doing it. As such, it is possible for anyone, anywhere at anytime to be mindful. However, mindfulness is more than *just* awareness of the present moment. It can be described as a *supercharged* awareness that is fully directed to the present moment in a non-reactive and non-judgemental way. As such, it is calm, curious and compassionate. In this chapter we will:

- Explore the meaning of mindfulness
- Explain how it is much more than *just* 'being aware', and define what it means to have a heightened awareness that is non-reactive and non-judgemental
- Explain how your innate capacity to be mindful can be enhanced by training
- Describe the benefits to body and mind of living mindfully

## What do we mean by mindfulness?

Mindfulness – the word, the concept – is everywhere these days, and seems to promise all things to all people. We find the word 'mindful' or 'mindfulness' connected to everything from gardening to therapy, sports coaching to computing. There are even mindfulness colouring books.

But is the mindfulness engaged in these varied activities all the same? Such broad use of the term has led to some confusion, as those excited by the promise of mindfulness attempt to navigate the wide range of offerings available. Exploring our understanding of what mindfulness really *is* in the pages that follow will help with this.

As well as being fully aware of what you're doing as you're doing it, mindfulness involves thinking about *why* we want to cultivate this awareness. This concept of intention is really important, as our intentions are the mental compass guiding all our actions. Why is being more present, more considered and more thoughtful important to you? This over-arching question is the key to unlocking your own unique mindful potential. Look at the Focus On box on page 22 to explore in more depth what most matters to you.

**Everyday usage of the word 'mindfulness'**

Many have struggled to find the words to adequately capture the richness of what it means to be mindful. After all, it's pretty difficult to describe an essentially non-verbal, sensory experience of body and mind. We do, however, use words relating to 'mind' and 'mindful' more than we realize in our everyday lives.

Have you ever borne someone's feelings 'in mind' when sharing news? When you do this you hold in mind the potential impact of your words on the other. You might deliberately

## FOCUSON EXPLORING WHAT
## REALLY MATTERS TO YOU

Depending on what is most important to you and
what you would like to change, you may approach
mindfulness in different ways. It is therefore worth
asking yourself the following questions and noting
down your answers:

- What made you pick up this book?
- What would you like to be different in your life?
- How much time and effort are you willing to put
  into making things different?
- What do you value most in life?

With your own priorities and intentions in mind, you will
use your mental and physical energy more wisely. You'll
be acting with awareness and in line with your most
heartfelt desires. Return to your answers periodically to
check they are still relevant as time goes by.

select words that will be less upsetting, for example, if you
are breaking bad news. Similarly, have you ever had to
'mind' the gap when getting on a train? If so, you have given
ongoing care and attention to your actions as you boarded

the train – to ensure you get home quickly and safely, which is your intention. And what about 'minding' your manners or your language in front of the kids? Same thing – knowledge or beliefs that help you fit in with the current cultural or social norms are held in mind to guide your actions and speech.

These three examples show that we all have the innate capacity to be mindful in its most basic form. Mindfulness, then, is when we become more aware of this capacity and/ or deliberately choose to develop it more deeply.

### A secular definition

Modern psychology has offered a variety of definitions of mindfulness. Most of them include a strong element of paying attention, without judgement to the present moment. Three of the most often cited definitions are:

*Mindfulness is paying attention in a particular way: on purpose, in the present moment, and non-judgementally.* (Kabat-Zinn, 1994)

*Mindfulness is the state of being attentive to, and aware of, what's taking place in the present.* (Brown and Ryan, 2003)

*Mindfulness is the non-judgemental observation of the ongoing stream of internal and external stimuli as they arise.* (Baer, 2003)

My own definition of mindfulness, based on 20 years of clinical experience, is 'awareness + 3'. To me, this means your ordinary awareness skills enhanced by being:

- fully directed to the present moment
- non-reactive (curious but calm)
- non-judgemental (compassionate)

It also works best when done in the service of something bigger (your over-arching intention) and with a particular attitude of kindness toward yourself (self-compassion). This definition captures *what* we are doing in the moment, *how* we are doing it, and the *why* that lies behind it.

Calmly accepting what happens to us, even when things are difficult, helps us to see clearly what is actually happening, not just what we think is happening. In this less volatile, less reactive mindset, we can make clearer choices about what to do next based on facts. We can see where we do have influence, and act in line with our bigger goals.

This doesn't mean passively accepting everything. It is an intention to be curious to learn more about how we relate to our minds, bodies, each other and the world. Learning is easiest if we are more compassionate and less critical and judgemental toward ourselves (and others) when mistakes are made. Without fear of judgement, we are more open and creative and can generate innovative solutions to life's challenges and obstacles because we learn how to be aware in a non-judgemental way.

## Why is the term 'mindfulness' still causing confusion?

Even having heard definitions of mindfulness, people often still get confused. Here are some reasons why:

- It sounds simple. But it's a lot harder than it sounds when we try to do it.
- We intend to be present, non-reactive and non-judgemental, but we find we are more often distracted, reactive and critical (of ourselves and others).
- We expect it to be quick, and yes, we all have the capacity to drop into the present moment at any time. Yet, the deeper transformative potential of mindfulness takes patience and persistence. It's not a quick fix.
- We are used to thinking about things using our conceptual, intellectual minds. As such, we have lost much of the ability to connect to our intuitive knowledge. This comes from directly sensing rather than consciously 'thinking about' what we, or our bodies, are doing. Having a 'gut feeling' about someone or something is one example of this.
- In our rush to 'get mindful' we often don't consider the intention that underpins our activity.

## What mindfulness is not

It is also important to consider what mindfulness is *not*. It is not the same as relaxation or 'zoning out'. Mindful awareness – mindfulness – requires your brain to be active and engaged, not spaced out or 'empty' of all thoughts.

Also, for the purposes of this book, mindfulness is distinct from meditation. This is because it provides the tools to allow you to use your mind flexibly and to its best potential, whether you're meditating, creating or relating to others. It is the building block that allows you to do any of these things, only better.

## Are awareness and mindfulness the same thing?

This is a complex question. As already touched on, awareness and mindfulness are related yet distinct concepts. Earlier, we described mindfulness as a type of *supercharged* awareness of the present moment. This, in turn, expands our awareness of our environment, body and mind, allowing us to discover things that were there all along, outside of our ordinary awareness, which previously never made it onto our radar.

We become more aware of our habits and patterns of thinking, so we can work to change any old patterns we no longer need. We can do this best if our awareness is mindful (fully present, non-reactive and non-judgemental); it's harder when we are distracted, reactive and overly critical.

## Changing awareness to mindfulness

Changing our everyday awareness into a deeper, more meaningful mindfulness requires attention and practice. Our awareness of our bodies, for example, changes all the time but is not always mindful. Because of our neural set-up and evolutionary influences, we often become *aware* of things in the context of minimizing physical and/or psychological harm. For example, body awareness increases when we trip over a broken pavement. The changing circumstances and resulting pain in our toe bring our attention rapidly to our bodies. Yet, this awareness may not be particularly mindful.

In fact, our reaction to the stubbed toe could well take us *away* from the present moment. We might go straight to the future, thinking 'Will I be able to go dancing/walk the dog tonight?' or 'Who's to blame for this?' Or, we might get lost in the past, 'Why didn't I see that?' or 'Did anyone see me trip and look foolish?' If this happens, we are not fully present, as reactivity and judgement have taken over.

If, on the other hand, we are practising mindfulness in this moment, the mental reactivity and tendency to judge would be noted and managed. Depending on what was most important to you, you could choose to drop the reactivity and consider how to better direct your attention, such as assessing the damage to your toe and taking appropriate action. The whole experience would then be different. In fact, research has shown that 57 per cent of the unpleasantness of pain comes from the mental reaction to it, not from the pain itself. The same principle applies with painful emotional experiences. Awareness alone may not be enough to help you manage this, whereas mindful awareness, or *mindfulness*, will mean you can meet these experiences in a new, more helpful way.

## Is mindfulness a natural state of mind?

We all have a natural capacity to be aware of the present moment when we are doing certain deliberate things, such as moving our bodies, creating something or relating to others. We can also access such moments of awareness fairly easily when engaging in pleasant activities, such as walking in nature or interacting with animals. These kinds of positive activities hold our attention in the present moment in a 'pleasant' way, giving us a brief taste of mindfulness.

However, we often need more training to be more *fully* aware – or mindful – when things are not quite as we want them to be, whether it's something small, such as a cancelled train, or life's bigger disappointments, such as relationship breakdowns, serious illness, or coping with death. It's at times like this you will most benefit from having a supercharged awareness that is non-reactive and non-judgemental.

## Recognizing shifts in awareness

Let's explore what you are already doing, and how you might make some tiny tweaks with big impact to develop your awareness and shift into mindfulness. There are many moments in the day when your awareness automatically changes, such as stepping outside your front door or stopping to answer your phone. Embrace these as natural learning opportunities, without you needing to do anything differently. Actually, you do have to do one thing differently – you have to start to notice and pay attention as a change in your awareness occurs. Simply paying more attention in these moments, for example, noticing what happens when you become aware of something (positive or negative) that you weren't aware of before, will strengthen your 'awareness muscle'. Tune in to the tone of your internal voice as well and try to keep it positive, more 'oh, look...' rather than 'oh, no, my attention has shifted again.'

As well as taking more notice of the things that are already going on in our minds, we can decide to pay more attention in other kinds of everyday moments. For example, make a conscious decision to sense the movement the next time you lift a cup of tea to your lips, or the pleasure of getting into a freshly made bed, or really notice how you feel when you hug someone dear to you. Furthermore, paying more attention to moments when you react strongly (to a stubbed toe, missed bus or something unexpected) will also help you to understand more about your reactive and judging habits.

## How can mindfulness be enhanced by training?

Deliberate mindfulness training (see examples on pages 112–123) will help us if we want to prolong the time we are able to spend in a mindful mode and/or be mindful under pressure. Although each of us has the capacity to be mindful, we all have different starting points when it comes to how distracted we are (and why), how reactive we are (and why) and how judgemental we are (and why). We therefore each need to look carefully at our personal circumstances and mental habits if we want to learn how to enhance our natural capacity for mindfulness and make it our new way of being. Further help with this can be found in Chapter 4.

### Environmental barriers to mindfulness

When we try to be fully present and mindful, we rapidly discover that our modern lifestyle is working against us. Here are a few examples of how we easily fall into mindless modes of living and being. These are some of the areas of life where mindful attention will bear most fruit:

- At work and play we often strive for harder, faster, more. Mindful living invites you to go slower, do less and be gentle.

- Smartphones and laptops draw us into virtual worlds, sapping our attention and reducing our connection with, and awareness of, our body. Mindfulness asks us to reside more in our bodies, allowing us to harness all the rich information it shares with us, each and every moment.

- Multi-tasking is not, in fact, doing several things at once, but is the rapid switching between multiple tasks. Although helpful in some situations, as we have become overwhelmed with information from multiple sources (texts, social media and numerous apps), multi-tasking more often creates stress, increases errors and is inefficient. Mindfulness suggests we do just one thing at a time.

- Advertising and cultural pressures push us to act in ways that may not be helpful or healthy. Social media often promotes comparison and competition, rather than compassion. Mindfulness asks us to stop, pause and check our intentions before acting, making us less susceptible to external influences that may not have our best interests at their heart.

- The media, in general, orients our minds toward fear and uncertainty, keeping us on edge and overly concerned about our own personal safety. Mindfulness asks us to have a balanced view, including noticing more overtly when things are going well and deliberately promoting positive, more compassionate and connected states.

## Our personal barriers to mindfulness

Sometimes the reason we do not feel 'fully present' is not due to external factors such as technology, but because of what is going on inside our own minds. We all have different levels of distraction, reaction and self-criticism/judgement that we will need to work through if we want to live more mindfully. These three factors are the opposite of the present moment, non-reactive and non-judgemental qualities that mindfulness training helps us to develop.

When we start to become more aware of our own minds, we are often surprised at how distracted we are, even if we have turned off the phone and intend to sit quietly. Scattered attention has become our dominant mode of being. Some people, whether consciously or not, use distraction as a technique to manage difficult emotional states or challenging situations. For example, 'workaholics' often discover through mindfulness that their work has been masking an emptiness, which is exposed when 'just doing nothing'. Engaging with this is the route to creating a more balanced and healthy life.

Similarly, reacting needlessly to things we don't like takes up a huge amount of brain resources. Whether it's small irritants or major obstacles, when you are not automatically reacting you can harness your brain resources to think more flexibly and creatively about problems, and as a result end up worrying less and increasing your productivity.

Self-judgement is another habit that often acts as a barrier to mindfulness. 'Beating ourselves up' when we make a mistake or let someone down only takes us off into a loop of self-recrimination that means we won't have a chance to see clearly what has happened and learn from it. Dropping this self-critical inner voice is the first step to seeing how we can grow from our mistakes. Modern culture often rewards people with perfectionist tendencies, but these unrelenting standards can have a heavy personal cost, such as when they result in anxiety and depression.

Luckily, we can use mindfulness to become more aware of these habits of distraction, reaction and self-criticism. Ask yourself when you next see any of these three mental patterns: 'Is this helpful and healthy?' This is the entry point to doing something different, if you wish.

## What are the stages of mindfulness development?

As with any training, getting going with mindfulness (a 'training' of the mind) requires focus and commitment. But, as familiarity with your body and mind develops, rest assured, it will get easier. There is a forward progression with some definite training stages and plateaus. And yet it's important to remember that there is no fixed destination, no 'blissed out state' to be obtained or 'side step' from life that takes you into an altered state of consciousness. Mindfulness is about developing the quality of your experience, just as it is.

The pace of your progress will be determined by how much priority you give the activity. Basic mindfulness skills can be picked up quite quickly, but more persistence and patience will be required if you want to broaden and deepen this to an all-round mindful-living approach to life.

**The early stages**

Initially, just being aware of the impact of factors such as excessive multi-tasking and technology on your body and mind and doing some 'spring cleaning' of your habits – especially tech habits – will have a huge impact. For example, turning off your text and email alerts while writing reports or cooking the dinner will make it much easier to get the task done, as it will increase your attentional capacity, allowing you to work more effectively and also reduce stress.

**Sticking at it**

Going beyond basic awareness to become less reactive and judgemental requires perseverance as you will need to see old, unhelpful habits in action many times before you learn their signature moves and are able to do something different.

More dedicated training, such as undertaking mindfulness practice at set times every day or week, will also give you the skills to be mindful under more extreme conditions. You'll be able to think clearly, communicate well, and keep your sense of calm and confidence, even under pressure.

The brain networks that control attention and awareness of our bodies and minds are highly plastic, meaning they can be 'rewired' at any age. As with developing any muscle, the more we train, the greater the changes in the brain.

## Is mindfulness training for absolutely everyone?

The media have led us to believe that mindfulness is for everyone and everything. Fundamentally, I believe that the majority of people can benefit from learning to pay more attention and take more care of their thoughts, speech and actions. However, the conscious practice of mindfulness may not suit everyone, or it may not be right for some, right now.

Those whose present moment experience is very chaotic or intense, such as the recently bereaved or those in the middle of a major crisis or life event, are advised to go slowly. Paradoxically, though, a time of crisis may also be a time when dramatic transformation is most possible. Sometimes it's in the toughest of times that it becomes clear old habits are no longer working, and this can really motivate people to try something radically different. Some patients with chronic depression or anxiety have found mindfulness training to be a real help in combatting symptoms of their illness.

Those with a low tolerance for negative emotions (and perhaps using drugs or alcohol as coping strategies), or with enduring relationship difficulties or trauma are also advised to go slow with mindfulness or train with the support of a health professional. People with perfectionist tendencies and strong inner critics may also struggle (to begin with) to be less judgemental with themselves. However, with the right support, and a bit of forethought and planning, everyone has the potential to unmask their capacity to live mindfully. Picking the right time to start and the right people to support you will help.

## What are the main benefits of mindfulness?

Mindful living is when we bring our mindfulness skills into everyday life, for as much of the time as is possible. The benefits of turning our normal awareness into this kind of more sustained mindfulness include:

- Feeling ok, even when things are not as we want
- Remaining calm, even under pressure
- Being able to use your rational thinking brain more efficiently and flexibly

- Being able to access a different type of intuitive knowledge through sensing changes in your body and mind
- Being able to think *and* feel at the same time (not sacrificing one for the other as we often do)

Fundamentally, mindfulness can change how we relate to our body, mind and each other.

## Benefits for the body

Relating mindfully to our bodies means taking better care of our posture, diet, fitness levels and all other aspects of self-care and healthy living, including any injuries or illnesses we may acquire. In the case of chronic physical illness, reacting less and cultivating a mindful relationship with one's body means you are likely to increase your enjoyment of life, even if you still have unpleasant symptoms.

Learning to engage during mindfulness practice with all the senses in the present moment will enrich our experience of the sensory world around us. We will feel moments of real vitality and presence, the sun or wind against our skin, for example, or the joy of just walking. It's not easy to put these non-verbal experiences into words, but a common response from someone who has just re-tuned to their body through practising mindfulness is 'Wow, I didn't realize all this was going on!'.

Becoming more tuned into our bodies and learning how to release and relax into our being also means we can feel the full range of emotional states that make us human. We might, for example, acknowledge emotional upset that manifests as physical tension, and then be able to do something about this, therefore making us feel both physically and emotionally freer and more healthy.

**Benefits for the mind**
With mindfulness we spend less time 'reacting' and more time engaging with what is really going on in the present moment. The benefit of this is that we get the chance to problem-solve any challenging situations more promptly.

A mind that is less reactive will be calmer and more content, even in a crisis. So much of our distress comes from the way the mind reacts to our experiences, rather than the experiences themselves, so reacting less often and less severely will make a huge difference to even an unpleasant situation. Knowing and managing your inner critic in this way allows you to be more vulnerable, connect more with others and thrive no matter what the circumstances.

Coming to realize, through mindfulness, that your thoughts are simply sensations in your mind can greatly reduce unnecessary anxiety. Try to let go, rather than hold on tightly, when you are preoccupied with thoughts about things that haven't yet happened or things that have already passed. This will make you feel more focused and grounded. Being present and aware of what we are experiencing, as well as holding in mind what matters to us most, also helps to deepen our self-knowledge, which, in turn, allows us to get on better with others.

## Benefits in relating to others

There is no greater gift you can give to another than your full present-moment attention, and yet having time for this is becoming increasingly rare in our modern world. A powerful sense of connection is created when we listen to others with a focused, highly tuned mind and body.

With the enhanced attentional skills developed by mindfulness, you'll be able to pick up on subtle, non-verbal clues, such as tone of voice, posture, amount of eye contact and (often), more importantly, what's not being said. You'll also be able to discern and hold in mind the intentions, desires and even beliefs of others. This enhanced social awareness can really help you improve relationships in all kinds of areas in your life.

However, this enhancement of our connection with others will only be achieved by the very honest engagement with our own reactions, assumptions and expectations as we train our own awareness.

### In summary

Practising mindfulness helps us to increase the frequency of being fully present and engaged as we act in, and on, the world. It fine-tunes our ability to stay on track with activities that are in line with our over-arching intentions and values. We become aware of the wealth of data from our bodies, minds and hearts that we can use to guide us in this journey called life. You can start from any point and, as this book will show you, there are multiple options to choose from if you want to develop your mindful 'awareness muscle'.

The true benefits of mindfulness are often seen in the inevitable moments when we face adversity. How we manage these is the real measure of our time on earth. We all draw different cards in life when it comes to the levels of joy and suffering we encounter. However, we all have the capacity to choose how we react or respond to what happens to us. In the next chapter, we will dive deeper into what is actually happening in our brains during mindful moments. From this, it will become more clear what you need to do to enjoy many of the benefits you have just read about.

## TRYIT DEVELOP AN ALERT–RELAXED MODE

The exercise below is a simple one but can have a profound impact on how you feel. You can do it anywhere to facilitate what is called an 'alert-relaxed' posture – both in your body and in your brain. Repeat it regularly to see what it's like to spend longer in the 'alert-relaxed' mode in both body and mind.

- Sitting or standing, stay still and focus your attention so it is prioritizing bodily sensations, particularly those from the back and spine. What can you notice?

- Now elongate your spine, as if someone is pulling you up by the tips of your ears. Very slowly, without force, making a small effort, but not straining.

- Try to work out the minimum muscles necessary to hold your spine alert. What is the maximum you can release to relax, without slumping?

- Now you are alert but relaxed in the body. Over time, you'll see that this physical posture helps your mind be alert–relaxed too (neither too tense nor too lazy).

# CHAPTER 2
How does mindfulness
actually work?

We discovered in Chapter 1 that mindfulness can be described as a supercharged awareness that is present, non-reactive, non-judgemental and guided by our intentions. It orients our mind to what's important to us now, in this moment of our life. It keeps us on track and less disturbed when we are (inevitably) pulled off-track.

In this chapter, we look into your brain to learn about the neural and cognitive processes that are engaged as you actively develop your awareness muscle when practising mindfulness. You'll gain an understanding of the natural processes that occur in all our minds, and learn that, contrary to what we might think, none of us are too 'distracted', 'fidgety', 'busy' – or whatever other misconceptions we might have – to become more mindful. You'll also discover *how* training your brain will give you the benefits you have been reading about.

### What is actually happening when I'm being mindful?

Try asking yourself this question now and again: 'Where is my mind right now?' Often you might notice that your mind and body are not in the same place. You may be sitting at home but your mind is still at work. Equally, you may be sitting at your desk, but your mind is everywhere except on your work. By asking yourself this question periodically you will start to become familiar with the four brain states that characterize a fully present 'mindful moment'. These happen, in order, repeatedly, in a continual cyclical journey. They are:

**1** Paying attention (to the present moment)
**2** Becoming distracted (lost in the future or past)
**3** Noticing that your mind has wandered
**4** Refocusing your attention back to the present moment

Recognizing these four stages will allow you to stop having potentially unrealistic expectations of feeling constantly calm, focused and 'in the zone' when practising mindfulness. Increasing your ability to know which of these stages you are in at any given time will help you know what to do next if your intention is to be mindful. And yes, you did read correctly, mind wandering is absolutely part of this process. Your brain *will* get distracted, but recognizing and working with this is a key part of mindfulness – it's what you do next that counts.

There are two additional key concepts we will explore here that underpin the whole endeavour. They are:

- **intention** – knowing why we are doing what we're doing
- **self-compassion** – recognizing that our learning and development process will be easier if we are kind to ourselves while practising

## The 4-step 'mindful moment' cycle

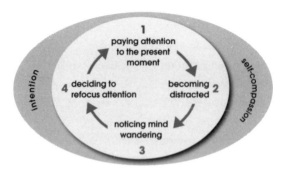

The diagram above illustrates the 4-step 'mindful moment' cycle that we will explore in this chapter. You'll see that the whole activity sits within the broader context of why we are doing this (our intention) and an attitude that promotes learning (self-compassion). It draws on both my own clinical experience and broader neuroscientific research, and I find that it really helps people understand how mindfulness works.

For those new to mindfulness, I hope this cycle will help you get acquainted with, and learn to recognize, the mind's normal 'mental movements'. For those who already have some experience of mindfulness training, I hope it will help to fine-tune an understanding of your practice, allowing you to move more skilfully back into the 'paying attention' mode when you realize your mind has been wandering.

The cycle is meant as a guide. The detail will emerge through your own exploration and practice. What is central is that you will be moving through these stages repeatedly during any attempt at mindfulness. This is how you will change your brain to transform your experience of your life. We'll also explore why fostering a kinder and less reactive awareness will accelerate your progress.

## What's my brain doing when I'm deliberately mindful?

Wendy Hasenkamp, a researcher in the field of mental health at Lesley University in the USA, has recently identified three brain networks that turn on and switch off as we move around the four stages of a mindful moment. These are called the **attention**, **default mode** and **salience** networks and they relate directly to my 4-step 'mindful moment' cycle, as follows:

**1** Our **attention network** is used to focus our attention on a selected object (for example, sensations related to breathing, sitting, walking or eating).

**2** Our **default mode network (DMN)** is activated when daydreams, memories or plans draw our focus elsewhere.

**3** Our **salience network** signals an alarm telling us our attention is no longer where we intended.

**4** We can then choose to re-engage our **attention network** to get back to the task of focusing on the selected object.

Going around the 4-step cycle is therefore like cross-training for your brain, as you are switching between brain networks the whole time (just as you'd switch between muscle groups in physical training). The more often you do this with awareness, the more you'll learn how these switches occur, the more you'll be able to control them and use your brain to its fullest potential, responding flexibly and appropriately in any situation. Use the exercise on pages 50–51 to try this out.

## How does my brain pay attention?

By choosing to focus our attention on a particular object, we engage our brain's **attention network**. Parts of this network can grow or shrink in response to how we use our attention in daily life. Some parts of it allow us to direct the spotlight of our attention where it is most useful, while another part, called the anterior cingulate, monitors whether our attention is where we decided to place it. With mindfulness, we 'train' this network so that we can more easily recognize the different characteristics of focused and distracted attention.

### What you pay attention to matters

When starting to practise mindfulness it helps to train your attention using objects that will most readily hold and capture it, such as movements, bodily sensations and the breath. These all have an in-built temporal quality that helps you to attend to the present moment as it unfolds. If you are focusing on an action such as breathing or walking, you can't, by definition, focus on the step or breath you took five minutes ago.

Although we are used to thinking that sensations are only from our bodies, in mindfulness, thoughts, memories and mental processes are also considered types of sensations. All of these arise, fade, can be attended to and ignored. Mental sensations are more abstract, subtle and slippery. This is why it's advisable we practise first with physical sensations. See the Focus On box on page 52 for more on the difference between physical and mental sensations and how to distinguish between them.

### Where you pay attention matters

When we look at a painting or watch a play we are aware of action in the foreground *and* the background. When we focus our attention on everyday things we similarly begin to notice what's in the foreground of our awareness (for example our breath), and what's in the background (perhaps sounds, or thoughts just outside of awareness). We can use our attention like a spotlight, moving it around to take in different parts of the internal or external scene, or we can narrow or widen the lens. These two features – foreground/ background and narrowing/widening – are important in the context of mindfulness, because *where* our attentional focus lies determines the information our brain receives. The narrowing and widening of attention can be deliberate or automatic. Narrowing the focus amplifies the signal, giving us more detail. This is helpful if we need to listen deeply in a conversation, but may be *unhelpful* if the focus of your attention is a worrying future thought or an unwanted pain.

## TRYIT ATTENDING TO THE BREATH

Many different objects – including the breath, movements, sound and, with a bit more practice, thoughts – can be used to train focused attention. Let's start for now with mindfulness of the breath, a popular and effective exercise.

It's just not possible to attend to a breath from the past or the future, as the breath is always in the present moment. Using your breath as your focus will allow you to see clearly when this focus is lost and your mind starts wandering, giving you the opportunity to bring it back to the breath with the help of the 4-step 'mindful moment' model.

1 Set your intention to attend to the sensations of breathing, labelling this 'breath'. Try to just observe your breath. Resist the urge to change or modify it.

Anything unexpected or unwanted (such as physical or emotional pain) naturally narrows the focus of our attention, as our brain is trying to tell us that something is wrong and needs attention. If, however, we have trained our attention using mindfulness, we have the option at these moments to

2 As best you can, **maintain the focus of your attention** on breathing, observing the impact of the air moving at the tip of your nostrils or into and out of your chest.

3 If **your mind wanders** (which it will, usually after just a few seconds), **note the distraction** and say to yourself 'this is not breath'.

4 Gently disengage from these 'not breath' sensations, no matter what they are – thoughts, worries, an itch, a niggling pain – and **re-focus attention** back to 'breath'.

You can do this for three breaths, or up to 300! As your attention skills develop, you'll be able to attend to more subtle sensations, and will likely find it easier to stay in the 'attention' zone for longer, and/or be able to return there more readily when you realize your mind has strayed.

## FOCUS ON DISTINGUISHING BETWEEN PHYSICAL AND MENTAL SENSATIONS

The hand-based exercise below will allow you to experience the difference between using *physical* movements and sensations, and *mental* sensations (thoughts and images) as an object of focus.

- Set your intention and posture in the alert-relaxed mode (see page 41). It helps to close your eyes.

- Place one hand on your leg or a nearby surface and focus your attention on the sensations as you lift your index finger up and down a few times. Then, try keeping the hand still and focus your attention on sensations from the still finger and the whole hand.

- Next, create and focus on an *image* of a hand in your mind, drawing from your memory your impressions of either your own hands or others.

If you are new to mindfulness, you are likely to find the physical sensations easier to stay focused on. But, with time, your ability to work with thoughts and visualizations will increase, so just keep practising.

re-widen our focus in order to see more clearly, put things into a broader context and note what wider choices or solutions are available.

**How you pay attention matters**

One of the key concepts in mindfulness is the word 'observe'. The trick is to simply 'observe' physical and mental sensations in a gentle, non-judgemental way as they arise. Remember the exercise on page 41 about being alert but relaxed in your body and mind? This means being alert to what's going on, yet relaxed in the sense that you're aware of receiving sensations but don't meddle with them or try to change them at all. You are looking, but not touching.

Why don't you try this right now with the breath, using the 4-step 'mindful moment' cycle on page 46. Take the basic breath exercise on pages 50–51 one step further by looking out for the precise moments that you move between the four steps (see the keywords in bold on that page for further guidance in this). As you do this, try not to be judgemental with your wandering mind. It'll be easier to get back to your intended task if you're calm and compassionate. Your brain muscles are being activated when you start to notice the changes between these four steps. And when you do this, fully in the moment and in a non-reactive and non-judgemental way, you are practising mindfulness.

## Where am I when my mind wanders?

Have you ever had to ask someone to repeat what they were saying to you because you were 'miles away' or 'lost in thought' and completely missed it the first time? These metaphors capture a universal experience of thinking our mind was in one place, only to be alerted (after the fact) that it was elsewhere. So where has it been?

A recent study suggests that we are not fully attending to what we are doing roughly 47 per cent of the time. Some of this mind-wandering is pleasant, some unpleasant. Some of it is directed by us, and some of it is automatic. Mindfulness helps us to study these movements and become more familiar with our own mental landscape.

## Your thinking, creating, wandering mind

As described on page 47, the default mode network (DMN) is the group of brain regions engaged during mind-wandering. When you are remembering, thinking, feeling, planning, analyzing, creating and imagining, you are using this network. If you become aware of any internal dialogue starting with the following words, your DMN is likely to be activated.

- If only... (remembering/analyzing – past reflections)
- What if... (creating/planning – future scenarios)
- As if... (imagining – possible scenarios/being elsewhere)

Or if you are a visual thinker you might experience mind-wandering in the form of images; a bit like an internal movie.

The DMN includes the hippocampus – the brain's memory region, which explains why mind-wandering can often involve memories. It also includes brain regions that allow us to imagine future scenarios (planning) as well as hold in mind others' thoughts and feelings (our emotional intelligence). DMN regions toward the back of the brain help us hold together a coherent sense of who we are (our sense of identity).

When we are doing boring or repetitive tasks, our DMN is often activated. One example of this is driving. It is all too easy to drive many miles barely noticing where we've been if we are preoccupied with thinking about something else. The DMN also likes to get busy when there is not much else happening, for example at night when we are trying to sleep. At such times we often become acutely aware of all the things 'on our mind', especially those we have been trying to avoid by keeping busy. As our mind flits forward and backward in time, these mental sensations capture our attention. If there are strong emotions involved, it can keep us awake all night. However, even simply becoming aware of such mental activity, choosing to disengage from thinking and focusing on the sensations in your body, the pillow, your pyjamas against your skin and the nice warm covers on top of you, is likely to calm the mind somewhat and may even relax you enough to enable you to finally drop off to sleep.

As seen on page 46, the wandering mind (your DMN) is a natural part of the 4-step mindfulness cycle, so it's important to learn to embrace it rather than fight it. Learning more about the positive and negative aspects of how your DMN is activated will increase your knowledge of your own mental habits.

### Positive mind-wandering

We are all familiar with the pleasant daydreams and fantasies that can capture our attention, pull us into an internal world and take us away from the here and now. There is certainly nothing wrong with savouring memories of a fun holiday or daydreaming about spending time with a loved one as happy thoughts tend to generate happy feelings. However, if you are using this strategy to manage low mood, or escape from unpleasant experiences, it may bring problems in the long term. It can compromise you at times when you need to be fully present, and if it becomes an engrained habit it can even prevent you from learning that you *can* tolerate difficult situations and that they will pass.

Having a busy, wandering mind can also be very useful in the creative process. We all have the capacity to imagine and play with thoughts, concepts and images in the service of innovation or problem-solving. As a mindfulness teacher, I am particularly interested in how the process of 'unclogging' the DMN through the conscious practice of mindfulness really opens up our creative potential. It's incredible to see, when teaching in the community, how many people reconnect with interests they have neglected since childhood when they start practising mindfulness, whether poetry, musical instruments, drawing, painting, dancing, singing ...

## Negative mind-wandering

But there are times when our mind-wandering can be very *unhelpful.* If we are, for example, planning, comparing or judging to excess, it can become very unpleasant. Or if we are stuck in an obsessive loop of thinking about something troublesome, it is likely to both impact on our mood and interfere with whatever other tasks we are doing. Knowing and being able to recognize these patterns, and particularly those that arise when things are not as we would like, is an essential part of the mindfulness process. We learn that these negative patterns of thought and behaviour are usually a reaction in response to our emotions and that we can actually *choose* just how 'reactive' we want to be. We always have the choice to pull back and say, 'Mind, I see you thinking hard about this issue for me. Thank you. However, this is not what I need to use you for right now.' With this gentle, compassionate awareness, and the intention to feel more positive again, you can disengage from the negative thought pattern, let go and come back to the present moment.

I encourage you to start naming these negative mental habits when you become aware of them, whether 'planning', 'judging', 'analyzing' or 'comparing'. A verbal label like this instantly disrupts negative DMN activity and puts you back in control by re-engaging your attention network (Step 4 of the 'mindful moment' cycle, see page 46). This process will involve you asking, 'Is this mental activity something I have chosen to engage in?' And then, 'Is it taking me toward or away from what is important to me?'

Although compelling, unhelpful thought loops are *not* your present moment reality and you *can* let them go (even though some may be kicking and screaming as you do so).

## How do I *notice* I've become distracted?

As we move through the 4-step 'mindful moment' cycle, we are now at Step 3: *awareness* of what our mind is actually doing when we realize that we've been distracted.

In the exercise on pages 50–51, you may have intended to focus on the breath but perhaps became aware at some point that you were thinking about emails, lunch, or even how great it feels to be mindful of the breath and how much you will practise in the future! Your brain's salience network, first mentioned on page 47, becomes engaged precisely at the moment you say to yourself, 'Oh, that's thinking about emails, not breath' (or whatever you had as the focus of your attention). Activation of this network is underpinned largely by the strength of your original intention to attend to the breath, which makes all 'not breath' sensations really stand out. Your brain is telling you that you have gone off-track and are no longer doing what you intended. It is then standing by, waiting for you to redirect it – you need to choose what to do next.

At this moment of awareness, we have the chance to spot some of our habitual reactions. In the breath exercise just mentioned, what happened to you when you realized your attention was no longer on the breath? How did you react to having 'failed' to stay focused? We each have our own unique reactivity patterns when unexpected things are brought to our attention. Commonly, our first reaction might be to judge ourselves harshly, or to start to analyse or compare. But mindfulness trains us to notice this and shift to responding in a calmer, more considered manner.

## How do I refocus on the present moment again?

To get back to the present as quickly as possible when you realize your mind has been wandering, it will help if you simply 're-mind' yourself of what you were doing, and why

## TRYIT NOTICING DISTRACTION

Using the breathing exercise on pages 50–51, experiment with different options when you notice your mind has wandered. Remember, you are (1) focusing attention, (2) going to get distracted, (3) noticing when this happens, and (4) trying to get back to the start. Don't worry if you go around and around the loop many times. The repetition *is* the mindfulness training, so practice will only improve your ability to move fluidly through the stages. Try out the following different options when you notice that you've become distracted:

1 Observe 'not breath' and go back directly. Don't give the 'not breath' sensations another second of attention, just recognize them as 'not breath' and get back.

you are doing it (your intention). This will be a lot easier and more pleasant if you can bring your attention back in a gentle yet firm way, rather than 'yanking' it. Disengaging from mental sensations is, on the whole, relatively easy if the thoughts are light and fluffy (for example, 'Hmm, what will I have for lunch?'). It's harder if more engrained or stronger emotions are driving the thinking. If you're afraid of flying, for example, it will be more challenging to let go of the thought

2 Allow yourself a quick look at the 'not breath' mental sensations. Don't hang around too long, though.

3 Engage more deeply with the 'not breath' sensations, watching your mind moving and gathering data about what's going on. Apply a verbal label, such as planning, analyzing, comparing, judging or doubting, before releasing and getting back to the breath.

4 Choose to stay with the 'non-breath' activity, whatever that may be, rather than go back. Make the distraction a new, intentional focus of your attention (rather than the breath). This option is often thought not to be mindful. However, if you deliberately intend and choose to follow a chain of thought, you are acting with awareness and it is mindful. You can then choose to come back to the breath at any point.

'What if something bad happens when I fly tomorrow?' The risk here is that we can be drawn into a secondary loop of distraction, involving berating ourselves for not being able to 'do' mindfulness. Don't worry, this is just another layer of emotional reactivity. Deal with it as before by gently telling yourself it's ok and reminding yourself what you were doing and why. As you go on to meet deeper, stronger patterns, more persistence, patience and practice will be required to get back to the 'present'. Just keep going; your efforts will be rewarded in the end.

## Why is there so much mention of intention?

We have explored two levels of intention so far. Firstly, we looked at the intention to focus on a certain object (for example, the breath or a body movement). Secondly, we considered the over-arching intention you had in mind when you thought about the 'bigger why' that underpins your interest in this topic (see page 22). In both cases, the intention informs all that follows. It operates behind the scenes, monitoring what unfolds moment by moment and alerting us when we go off track. But how does it do this?

Scientists have discovered a brain region that is responsible for preparing us for action. Before we have even moved, or are aware we will move, blood flows to this area and we can sense the urge or impulse to act. You can experience this for yourself the next time you are about to scratch an itch.

This region is engaged all the time, for example when walking. It helps your brain remember past experiences of 'walking' and creates a 'shimmer' in the mind of the anticipated sensations associated with walking, such as 'foot touching floor', 'leg swinging' and 'weight transferring'. These anticipated sensations are held in mind as the activity unfolds. As real-time sensory information enters the brain it is cross-checked against what was anticipated. If there is a match, we barely notice we are walking. If there is a mismatch, such as if we stumble or fall, the brain immediately makes us aware of it, so we can choose what to do next.

When we intend to focus on the breath the same process is involved. The intention sets up the expected sensations (air moving, lungs expanding, ribs moving, etc) against which the on-going real-time sensations are compared. When we start thinking 'tomorrow's meeting' or 'this weekend's party', our salience network taps us on the shoulder and says, 'Hello, I was expecting air moving, tummy rising and falling, and now I am getting tomorrow's meeting/this weekend's party and you rehearsing what you will say, is this right? Is this what you want me to do now?' – allowing us to decide whether to continue with the new thoughts or get back to focusing on the breath.

At the highest and most abstract level, our over-arching intentions direct our lives. When we can hold in mind what is important to us (our values) during our day-to-day activities (including our mindfulness practice), everything changes. We find we act, speak and think differently, and what we choose to do, or not do, changes. Moreover, we understand that the mind can be oriented toward our desires, without being wedded to a certain outcome. We can approach life in a directed, but flexible manner. This is mindful living.

## Why is self-compassion helpful?

You don't *have* to be kind to yourself in life, but it helps! If you really check and experiment, you'll discover that you learn faster if you are gentle with yourself when you make mistakes.

The moment of awareness during your mindfulness training that your mind has wandered is the place where you can practise non-judgement. So, instead of saying, 'Oh ****, I am not on the breath,' modify your inner dialogue to have a softer, less judgemental tone: 'It's ok, I see you, distraction, you are welcome, but not now, I'm on the breath, thanks.'

Mindfulness is all about learning how we relate to our experiences. Whether facing everyday stressors or life's major challenges, practising self-compassion will lessen your automatic judgemental reactions and increase the chances of acting thoughtfully and constructively.

## Using judgement skilfully

'Is it *always* a bad thing to judge?' is a common question mindfulness students ask and, of course, the answer is no. In your own values system, there will be things you consider 'right' and 'wrong', and this is important. In mindfulness, however, you are being asked to check if that moment is an appropriate time to engage the judging process. Judging yourself harshly for feeling an emotion or making a mistake is rarely helpful. As with all mental processes, choosing *when* to judge is the skill that mindfulness develops.

## So, why is practice important?

With continued practice you will become more familiar with the 4-step 'mindful moment' cycle and therefore more experienced at detecting the mental movements of your own mind. You will be able to focus your attention on any object (or task) for longer, be less impacted by distractions and learn from your mistakes. The new way you are relating to yourself will spread out to your relationships with others (see page 39), enriching your experience of being in the world.

## Types of practice

You can practise mindfulness informally – wherever you are, at any time – or formally, which means dedicating some regular time to practise, perhaps after attending some mindfulness classes to get you going.

Anything from walking and running, to listening and eating can be conducted 'mindfully' as what I like to call 'informed informal practice' if they are done holding the 4-step cycle (see page 46) in mind. Make it your intention to do only that one activity, then notice when your mind wanders; don't react or judge, and choose to come back to the start.

If you want to go deeper, or have met some unruly mental habits that you feel need more work, a regular formal practice is advised. For this, you'll need to dedicate time to practise, and do so in conditions that will maximize your efforts. Turn to Chapter 4 for some guidance on this. Remember, it's not about creating blissed-out states, practising only when you feel good or avoiding what's going on in our minds. The real power of mindfulness is seen in exactly those moments when everything is going wrong, we feel we can't cope and we want to run and hide.

**Advantages of practice**

Whether you decide to try formal or informal practices, if you engage your mindfulness brain network repeatedly, things in your life *will* start to change. Among other things, you will:

- become more in tune with your body and mind
- increase control of your capacity to focus and stay in the present moment
- become less emotionally reactive, therefore feeling generally calmer and more balanced
- develop your emotional intelligence

- understand and directly experience the power of self-compassion and kindness
- increase the time you spend daily in the mindful mode

**In summary**

Setting your intention, understanding the bigger why and being gentle and kind to yourself are the foundations for an effective mindfulness practice. Within that, start with any activity that will allow you to identify the 4-step 'mindful moment' cycle and give your brain a good workout. Remember, however, that mindfulness is not a static destination, but an ongoing journey, and that you will continue to learn and grow the more you practise.

The key is flexibility, being able to choose where to direct your brain's incredible resources. We already have the neural machinery in place, ready to work for us. As we shall see in Chapter 3, humans have long been interested in developing the supercharged awareness that is mindfulness. As you read on, you will find out how to do this for yourself in the modern world, but let's turn now to the origins of mindfulness.

# CHAPTER 3

Where does mindfulness
come from?

In the previous chapter we discovered that the neural circuitry we need for mindfulness is already there, in our brains. Everything is ready to go, but how easily we can access it depends on a variety of factors. Mindfulness is a quality of presence that's innate and yet we can also train it. The origins of mindfulness are, therefore, both genetic and environmental. In this chapter we will explore:

- How awareness and mindfulness are in our genes
- How humankind has attempted to investigate awareness and mindfulness
- How some traditions have developed detailed roadmaps of how to train awareness and transform it into mindfulness
- The modern manifestations of mindfulness

## Is mindfulness in our genes?

We humans have a unique capacity to be aware of both what we, and, to a large extent, others, are thinking and feeling. This has enabled our species to live in large social groups, become less preoccupied with survival than other animals and, therefore, more able to dedicate brain space to planning, innovating and creating.

### Awareness is in our genes

One theory suggests that our brains, and particularly our massive frontal lobes, developed to help us meet the demands that arose when we started living together, given that this requires so much awareness, care and sensitivity in order to foster a harmonious environment. We developed brain networks that allow us to mentally explore the past, future or mind of another. It's part of our evolution.

## The double-edged sword of awareness

However, what was once helpful may be less so today, as our external world has evolved at a rate much faster than our brain. And trying to keep our brains going as fast as everything around us can harm us. For example, excessive reflecting, comparing and judging is leading to an epidemic of low mood. Statistics from the World Health Organization suggest that depression will be the largest health burden on society by 2030. Similarly, excessive planning, controlling and worry are ingredients for anxiety. We can completely clog up our brain networks with past and future activity that isn't 'real', making us blind to the present moment. Not only does this mean that we might miss valuable information that could help us in that moment, but it also adversely affects our ability to really connect and empathize with others.

Despite the potential pitfalls, self- and other-awareness is still vital for our survival, even in today's modern age. There are multiple routes to develop self-awareness, and humans have always been curious about how to do this.

## How have we expanded our awareness?

Humans have always tried to expand awareness through various means, including taking spiritual, self-developmental, creative and chemical paths, each of which we will look at briefly in the text that follows. These activities, whether they take the form of a yoga class, therapy session or prayer practice, often tap into the brain networks described in the 4-step 'mindful moment' cycle (see page 46) and have some common touchpoints with mindfulness – acting with care, paying attention, being non-judgemental and compassionate. However, it is important to recognize that their methods can differ slightly in relation to their over-arching intentions.

If you have explored your awareness via any of these routes, the good news is that you are likely to have already trained some of the relevant neural networks for mindfulness. However, watch out if your mind gets caught up in comparing your yoga/therapy/prayer practice to what you are learning in mindfulness. There are similarities, but important distinctions:

### Spiritual paths

Many spiritual and religious practices engage the mindfulness brain networks to train awareness. The intention is to connect to divinity – however this is defined. There is usually an ethical framework to support this development of awareness, based around taking care of self and others.

Religious training is often through repeated prayers or rituals, contemplative exercises, periods of silence and retreats. Monastic and contemplative communities, for example, have studied for centuries the best ways to train awareness. It's hard to say your prayers if your mind is cluttered with 'to do' lists, or worries about parking tickets. If the mind wanders off, it is better if you can notice promptly, and get back to the task of prayer. Sound familiar? You are moving around the 4-step cycle as you do this. Your focused attention is on the prayer. As such, mindfulness training can augment faith practices. Indeed, some of my clients say mindfulness has increased their focus during prayers and their ability to stay close to their spiritual intentions.

A feature that often permeates spiritual practices is the belief that the divine (in whatever form) has a loving and supportive attitude, no matter what. However, students from some faith backgrounds can encounter strong judgemental habits if, for example, they have been encouraged to carefully monitor thoughts and feelings, checking they are in line with the teachings that they follow. If some thoughts are considered 'right' and some 'wrong', it can lead to reactive and critical engagement with the mind, which can, in turn, become a generalized, widely applied habit. Mindfulness encourages a calm but curious non-reactive discernment, rather than automatic judging.

## Self-development paths

Psychologists and other therapists have explored ways to develop awareness for many years. This has been with the intention of healing emotional wounds, building self-esteem and shining a light on unhealthy relating habits. There are multiple routes, each with a slightly different emphasis on where the healing occurs. Research has shown, however, that the type of therapy you do is not the most important factor. Rather, it is the expectation that something can be different and the relationship with the therapist that are key to success in therapy.

Being held in mind by someone who is paying you deep and consistent attention in a non-reactive and non-judgemental manner has been found to be what allows you to work best through painful memories and emotions. A therapist who uses a type of mindful awareness helps *you* to develop a similar awareness, and to start to embody for yourself new ways of thinking and feeling.

## Creative paths

Humans have always tried to find ways to share important experiences through the arts, and exposure to art helps us to connect to the core of the human condition – our emotions. Great art, whether music, dance, painting or sculpture, provokes us to feel and think in new ways, expanding our

## FOCUS ON RECOGNIZING MINDFULNESS IN OTHER AREAS OF LIFE

Think about anything you do regularly that you believe is mindful, such as yoga, prayer or therapy sessions. Keep in mind that mindfulness is simply being aware of the present moment, in a non-reactive and non-judgemental way, in the service of larger intentions, and think through the 4-step 'mindful moment' cycle. When you next do the activity, ask yourself:

- Is your body and mind in the same place during the activity? Or has your mind wandered off task?

- Are you intending to attend to the present moment? Or are you on autopilot, going through the motions?

- Are you monitoring your focus, noticing when you are losing it and taking deliberate action to get back?

- Are you alert to any judging and reactivity in the mind and actively managing this in a mindful way?

- Are you being gentle to your body and mind?

awareness. If we can engage with art in a non-judgemental, non-reactive and present moment manner, we will be able to connect to the message and intention of the artist in a more meaningful way.

## Chemical paths

Across human history chemical means have been used to alter awareness for various intentions. The shamans of Latin America and elsewhere use plant-based hallucinogenics to journey into altered states where deep personal and spiritual insights can arise. Similarly, artists and musicians have also long experimented with natural and manufactured chemicals to open up awareness and see beyond our conditioned minds. These chemicals influence the same brain networks that we engage with mindfulness. And in the medical field there is now clinical research being conducted into the use of some chemicals, such as ketamine and LSD, to treat various mental health conditions.

This route to expand awareness is not for everyone. However, knowledge on how to access deep insights in a short period of time is of interest to those in healing professions. How these insights are retained remains a question. For reliable and lasting effects, many argue that the discipline of routine daily practices cannot be replaced. It is via repeated, directed attention that we can most reliably transform neural networks.

## Does mindfulness come from Buddhism?

Of the traditions that have really honed 'roadmaps' to mindful awareness, Buddhism has done so most thoroughly. Developed and refined over the centuries, Buddhist mental training techniques are a very clear path to develop the specific type of awareness that is mindfulness (present moment, non-reactive and non-judgemental).

### The Buddhist connection

In Buddhist traditions dating back to the 5th century BC, mindfulness training is a foundational skill, the overarching intention of which is to gain mastery over the mind in order to reduce suffering for all beings (including the self). Mindfulness in this context supports many more advanced Buddhist practices (including those that train attention, insight, visualization and heart-centred exercises). Yet, it is also in and of itself a very powerful awareness development process.

The specificity and detail of the Buddhist path to develop mindful awareness naturally appeals to Western scientific minds who are now studying this topic with renewed interest. This has led many to believe that mindfulness comes solely from Buddhism. However, it is not the only origin. In fact, Buddhist thought itself was informed by earlier Indian thinking, and a number of other ancient civilizations also investigated how to develop mindful awareness.

### The philosophers' connection

Mental exercises similar to those found in Buddhism can be found in Western Classical antiquity, from the philosophers of Ancient Greece and Rome. Pythagoras (c. 580–500 BC) encouraged mindful reflection on the day's activities, to check if one's actions were in line with one's intentions. The school of Epicureanism (4th-century BC) developed exercises to help people notice when 'mental proliferation' (the mind getting carried away with itself) occurred, with the aim to reduce the distress this mental activity creates in daily life. The Stoics (3rd-century BC) promoted present-moment attention (referred to as prosochē), as part of daily exercises for learning the truth about the self and the world. And a later Stoic, Seneca (4 BC–65 AD), encouraged exercises to increase the stability of the mind, and to investigate whether thoughts arise intentionally or automatically. Ultimately, the intention of these exercises was to manage our mind to help us live well and in harmony with one another. They demonstrate how Western traditions of thought developed awareness in a similar way to Eastern traditions, and for broadly the same intent.

### Where does modern mindfulness come from?

In our modern culture, mindfulness has once again emerged. This time, it's presented within a Western healthcare context but is expanding rapidly. Framed in scientific language backed up by research, modern mindfulness derives largely from the Mindfulness Based Stress Reduction (MBSR) programme created by Jon Kabat-Zinn at the University of Massachusetts in the 1970s, variations of which are now found worldwide.

## Mindfulness reinvented in healthcare

The intention of MBSR was to help people with chronic pain manage their illness. Stress, including mental agitation and struggle, was found to exacerbate physical symptoms. Using mindfulness techniques to develop a non-reactive, non-judgemental awareness of pain was found to be helpful for pain management. Now, more than four decades of research shows that MBSR also improves quality of life, psychological and physiological functioning, and the ability to relate to oneself and others. Mindfulness can even change how our immune system functions and may impact on factors related to aging.

The recognized standard eight-week MBSR course involves 2 hours' group practice per week plus a home practice of 45 minutes per day. The course offers a mix of various exercises, education about stress and chronic illness, and training in self-care. Although presented as a secular training, with reference to spiritual/religious elements removed, Kabat-Zinn openly describes how he drew on his own spiritual path (Zen Buddhism) to inform the practices and protocol. This approach has helped make mindfulness accessible to hundreds of thousands of people, including many with chronic illnesses, whose lives have been incredibly transformed.

### Integrating body and mind

The success of the MBSR programme really reminded those who work in physical health about the impact of the mind on the body. A related programme, based on MBSR but adapted to reduce the likelihood of relapse into depression, is Mindfulness Based Cognitive Therapy (MBCT). This was developed by research clinicians John Teasdale, Zindel Segal and Mark Williams at Oxford University in the 1990s. The team discovered that paying attention to the body and learning to tolerate emotions, as well as learning the unhelpful habits of mind that perpetuate low mood, are the keys to this. Developing the attentional skills to nip these habits in the bud helps to prevent downward spirals of thinking. Research indicates that an attitude of self-compassion, and the experience of the facilitator or trainer, are also key elements.

Mindfulness is now found in physical and mental health services worldwide, predominantly, but not exclusively, in the form of these two programmes, MBSR and MBCT (or variations on them). Western medical tradition has long separated physical and mental health, to the detriment of patients. Now, with mindfulness providing a route to join mind and body, new truly holistic and integrated healthcare is possible.

## An explosion of interventions

Results from the MBSR and MBCT programmes seen in healthcare have piqued the curiosity of pretty much anyone interested in improving attention, creativity, emotional intelligence and problem-solving in any setting.

Mindfulness in schools is just one example of its increasing popularity as there is a real recognition that children need help with emotional well-being. There's also an understanding that as facts and knowledge become available at the click of a button, the skills young people need for future success are the social and emotional skills that will help them to work in multi-cultural, multi-lingual, trans-global environments.

## Some issues with modern mindfulness

As mindfulness has rapidly gone mainstream there have been several concerns, however. On one side are those from contemplative traditions who believe that mindfulness has been simplified, stripped of its ethical framework and, as a result, is not the real deal. On the other hand, there are those who believe that what is being taught is 'Buddhism by stealth'. They are worried that intentions are not clear and that asking children to 'meditate' in school, for example, is not appropriate. There is no doubt that people are experiencing the benefits of mindfulness; the problems are more in relation to what it is called, where people think it comes from, and lack of clarity and communication about the over-arching intentions. Clearly, spending five minutes focusing attention on your posture is not the same as a life-long commitment to Buddhist practices. However, 45 minutes practice per day for eight weeks can start to shift your perspective and orient your mind toward being a bit gentler to yourself and others. Is this Buddhism, or re-connecting to our innate, evolutionary story?

The neuroscientific findings around mindfulness continue to create excitement. However, what we discover in the brain is often just confirming what's been reported in the spiritual traditions for millennia. It provides a modern-day 'convincer' that appeals to the Western intellectual mind in a language that is friendly and non-threatening, yet ultimately opens the door to the same paths that have been explored by our ancestors. This surely suggests that mindfulness is a core human experience, rather than something reified in one tradition or another.

### In summary

Finally, for now it is important to remember the fact that if you keep practising mindfulness, things *will* change – you are stepping onto a 'path' of sorts. And, despite the fact that, in secular mindfulness, this path has not been fully elaborated in the same way it has in the spiritual traditions, it has been shown that if you keep practising, your awareness will broaden and deepen. You'll start to meet experiences that are well defined in spiritual trainings but less well understood (for now) by Western psychological and medical models. This is all part of the learning, about yourself and others, that comes with mindfulness and, with continued practice, you will start to enjoy the physical and emotional benefits of mindfulness as described in Chapter 1.

My top tip for engaging in mindfulness is to approach the endeavour with playfulness in your heart. There is no single 'right' way to do this, and finding something that engages you and is fun to begin with will set the right tone for your training. You may meet challenges, but working through them is the work to be done with mindfulness. Try to keep things light and not get too serious about it all. In the process, your experience of yourself, including the notion of 'self', and the world will change, and you will find yourself more resilient, empathetic and adaptable than you perhaps thought possible.

# CHAPTER 4

How can I get the most
out of my mindfulness?

As with any training, if you want to access the benefits of mindfulness, some effort is involved. A little preparation will therefore stand you in good stead and ensure that your time, effort and money are wisely spent. While we all have an innate capacity to be mindful, some dedicated thinking and planning will really pay off if you want to enhance your mindfulness. In this chapter we will look at:

- How to prepare for mindfulness training
- How to be mindful in mindless environments
- Personal factors that may impact on your practice

Having done this preliminary thinking, you will find the whole experience of engaging with mindfulness much more, well, mindful. You will already be acting with awareness, giving care and attention to your situation, and ensuring you are using your energy as intended.

## How can I best prepare to start mindfulness training?

There are many ways to supercharge your awareness into the present-moment, non-reactive, non-judgemental awareness that is mindfulness. Apps, books, workshops and courses can all develop mindfulness and train your brain. And when you looked at your motivation in Chapter 1 (see page 22), you started the preparation that will help you select the route that works best for you, no matter what your starting point.

## Finding time for mindfulness practice

Mindfulness training is fundamentally about learning to care for ourselves, which, sadly, is rarely a priority in our busy modern lifestyles. Reflect for a moment on your timetable last week. How many of your activities were nurturing? How many were depleting? How quickly did you set aside activities that 'fill the tank' (such as going to the gym, seeing friends, resting) as work projects ran over, others needed you, or something unexpected blindsided you? The ironic truth is that things that help us cope when the pressure is on are often swept aside just when we most need them. These are exactly the times to pause, gather our thoughts and make time for them.

How badly you want things to change will dictate your approach to mindfulness. Formal dedicated practice requires your full attention, selecting a programme of study and sticking to it – just like choosing to learn a language. if you're still not sure you are ready to commit to this, then weaving informal practices into your daily life may allow you to test out how mindfulness can work for you.

A common complaint is 'I don't have time to practise'. Think about your current timetable and be realistic. Can you fit in formal practice and what might you need to let go of to make space? It's rarely that we don't have time. It's that we are not valuing or prioritizing the activity enough to make time for it.

### Being flexible

When considering practices it's counterproductive to be too rigid. Give whatever you choose a good try, but if something is really not working it is sensible to pause and reconsider. Remind yourself of your larger intention and see if you can be more flexible. The changes in the brain that lead to ever-increasing mindful awareness are directly related to the number of times you engage and disengage the

---

#### FOCUSON DETERMINING THE BEST ROUTE FOR YOU

**Informal training:** For busy parents, workers and those caring for others, informal training is appealing as it needn't add anything to your schedule. Practices can be done anywhere, anytime, and provide a testing ground to get a sense of your natural (dispositional) mindfulness abilities. Reminders on your phone, diary, stickers or screen-savers can prompt you to practise and help shore up your intention to do so. Bearing in mind the 4-step 'mindful moment' cycle on page 46, focus on:

- Mindful communication (see page 122) in every conversation. This will hone your attentional skills and allow you to learn more about your wandering mind.

brain networks described in Chapter 2, so there really is no substitute for actual practice. Sometimes, however, it's just not possible to practise.

So, what else can you do that will still move you in your desired direction? Perhaps read a book, watch a video, or Google 'mindfulness' and see all the weird and wonderful ways that mindfulness is being used worldwide.

• Mindful walking (see page 112) – my personal favourite. You'll be training your brain every time you walk to your car, to the bus stop or up the stairs.

**Formal practices:** These mean a commitment to practise at a dedicated time for a dedicated length of time. Pick a time (for example, a specific night during the week), a duration (start with 5–10 minutes and work up to 25–40 minutes) and a practice (see Chapter 5 for suggestions) and do it, no matter what. Research shows that we break and make habits in 30 days. Give yourself the chance to experience the effects of regular mindfulness practice. One good idea is to make yourself accountable to a friend who can support you, and to reward yourself with a treat if you manage to achieve what you intended.

I initially ask some clients to do anything they find pleasing and nurturing for just five minutes a day. This acclimatizes them to making time for themselves, without the pressure of 'having to do' mindfulness or adding mindfulness to an already heaving to-do list. What would you choose? A walk through the park, drinking a cup of your favourite tea, or listening to a piece of music you love? Then make that activity something you do mindfully, and eventually turn it into a formal practice slot. Start small, don't be too rigid and make self-care your primary intention.

**Finding the right place to practise mindfulness**

The word mindfulness often evokes an image of a blissed-out yogi, sitting cross-legged, eyes closed in a beautiful natural setting. You definitely don't have to be seated like this to be mindful! Closing your eyes does help to minimize distractions, but it's not essential. Isolated locations are optimum for focused attention training as there are fewer distractions (sounds, visitors, arguing neighbours, etc.), which means you can train your attention on the more subtle sensations of body and mind, and learn more quickly. However, for those of us who need to get started in the real world, it helps to take time to think about some alternative places to practice. Ideally, find a space where you will be undisturbed for a set period. You might try a local library, a church or a gallery if you are struggling to find a quiet place at home or work.

If your mindfulness training is in a noisy environment, maybe next to a fire station or a school, for example, it is likely to be tough for beginners. I once ran a group that had a samba band practising next door. It turned out, however, that for those with a bit more experience, wanting things to be different in that moment ('Don't they know we're meditating here?!') provided a great opportunity to develop the non-reactive quality of awareness.

**Being mindful in mindless environments**

For many working adults, the majority of their time is spent in environments that are far from mindful. Indeed, they are often in places that foster distraction, reaction and criticism. We know from increasingly alarming statistics that people around the world are suffering both mentally and physically from the demands of modern working conditions. Across all sectors, people are being asked to do more for less and this often means the work/life balance is compromised. Mindfulness is desperately needed but can seem totally impossible in these situations. Yet, some small, deliberate changes, such as learning to pause, acting with intention and listening to our bodies, may be very helpful.

In some organizations, mindfulness is offered to help those whose working conditions are inherently stressful (medics, air traffic controllers, military), and for those who want to think more deeply and creatively. The research on the benefits of mindfulness at work is compelling. Organizations that make time in the day for mindfulness have been proven to have happier, more productive and more innovative staff. However, for those who are already over-stretched and time-poor, more creative mindfulness training options are used. The work I do with healthcare staff, for example, focuses on weaving mindful moments into their day, such as doctors practising mindful walking as they collect their patients from the waiting room. If you are really stuck, I cannot emphasize enough how just getting outside and breathing fresh air will get you part way to the present moment with very little effort. Research has shown that even looking at pictures of nature improves our attention, so take advantage of your lunch/tea breaks and explore any green spaces nearby.

Even a drop of mindfulness in a mindless environment will shine like a beacon of light. Others around you will become curious when they see you are less 'headless chicken' and able to be curious, connected and creative even in challenging moments.

**Other considerations**
One thing we know helps when learning mindfulness, as with any new skill, is having someone on your side to motivate you and help you keep going, so think about who could be a mentor or supportive friend for you. You might also consider:

- Finding a group of mindfulness practitioners (or even a Meetup/Facebook or other online group)
- Seeking out new environments to meet like-minded people
- Reviewing how much time and energy you spend doing things in line with your values (or not)
- Taking time out of your usual setting so you can plan and design a practice regime

## What personal factors can impact mindfulness?

Some fairly predictable hurdles will be encountered when we turn our attention to the space of the mind. This section will help you understand how your mind may impact on or react to your efforts to be mindful. For example, how you've used your brain in the past, some of your personality traits and how you relate to your emotions are all relevant. Your ability to move around the 4-step 'mindful moment' cycle shown on page 46 will be made easier if you take the time to explore your unique mental profile. Just as an athlete might complete a body type and gait analysis in order to design a personalized training programme, so you can determine your optimum training experience and get the most out of mindfulness with this preparation.

Taking time to do this preparatory work can feel annoying initially, as you may be used to starting things immediately. But, in mindfulness, we are aiming to undo some of our less helpful habits. Let's look at how you regularly use your mind.

## Different experiences create different mental habits

Research has shown that similar groups of people tend to be susceptible to some similar mental habits that can impact on their mindfulness practice. For example, people who spend a lot of time in nature are often more inherently mindful, as the external environment holds their attention. However, when they are asked to focus attention just on the breath, for example, and need to rely on *internal* attentional resources, they can struggle.

Artists are often familiar with many techniques that explore attention and creativity. They are adept at letting their minds wander but they, too, can struggle to bring focused attention to something more mundane such as the soles of their feet.

Those who have studied psychiatry, psychology, coaching or any other training that involves understanding other minds have also usually fine-tuned their awareness in a certain way. They tend to have trained strong habits to analyse, compare and interpret. When attempting mindfulness they often get stuck in the conceptual 'thinking about' habit, and find it hard to just 'sense' without elaborating or working out why.

When I have worked with medical professionals I have observed a different kind of common obstacle, particularly with mindfulness of the body. Because they have trained for years to understand the anatomy and function of the body, they automatically bring up visual imagery and facts when they focus attention on the body. It's vital for their work and we don't want them to stop doing this. However, this neural activity is additional to what's being asked of them during mindfulness, which is the direct observation of raw sensory information (no pictures or thinking required). Physical trainers and anyone else with highly visual minds may also experience this. It's not wrong, it's just a different use of your brain. Letting go of well-practised habits like this during formal mindfulness training will increase your ability to use your awareness more flexibly. Remember, the brain is highly plastic – anything we do repeatedly will change its wiring.

## The impact of personality traits

Some common personality traits can work against you if you are trying to become more mindful. If you recognize some of the tendencies described in the text that follows, don't panic. You can still develop mindfulness; knowing about these obstacles upfront will simply help you recognize them when they occur.

Many of us have strong perfectionist tendencies, which can get in the way of supercharging awareness in a non-reactive and non-judgemental way. Striving to get everything right by evaluating performance is a valued trait in our society, and often associated with success. Yet there are costs to this way of thinking and living. When these traits are active and operating without awareness, it can lead to burnout and exhaustion.

There are also those who have a natural tendency for avoidance – whether of conflict, distress or negative emotions – which can make mindfulness challenging in a different way. Avoidance can be behavioural (for example, avoiding difficult or fearful experiences), cognitive (drifting off into sleepiness or daydreaming) and/or linked to addiction (food, drugs, alcohol, media, sex, etc). Perhaps this was helpful when other coping strategies were not available. However, mindfulness asks us to be open, curious and interested, rather than look away from the source of our suffering.

Many come to mindfulness because they are starting to have an inkling that these coping strategies have disadvantages. For one, they take up a lot of energy. Being busy avoiding something can give a false sense of dealing with the problem. In fact, it often means we are unable to see clearly what's really going on, and miss valuable information that can help us see where we might make positive changes. This is misapplied mental energy that gives power to the very thing we are attempting to control. Critical here is to engage with the mind with persistence, patience and compassion. Underneath avoidance can sometimes be a deep sense of loss or feelings of unworthiness or incompetence. This may be

unmasked when we stop avoiding and can be painful.
But it is through the gentle engagement with the habit and
the underlying wounds that we can gain real freedom.

**Vulnerability takes strength**

Mindfulness asks us to be gentle as we relate to our thoughts,
feelings and bodies. This really is the best way to learn, but
many of us find this surprisingly difficult. Some associate being
gentle with being weak or passive. Men, in particular, tend to
need convincing that being kinder to themselves when they
experience emotions is helpful. It goes against our cultural
narrative of what it means to be a 'man'. And yet, the fact
that suicide is the leading cause of death for men under 50
in the UK, and the second leading cause in the US, clearly
indicates there is a dire need to help change the habit of a
'stiff upper lip'. The evidence is clear that mindfulness can
prevent depression and is one way to help all of us respond
differently when feelings of hopelessness and isolation arise.

Perfectionists believe if they let up on themselves for one
second, they won't achieve anything. This assumption
warrants investigation. One student of mine with these
tendencies eventually had a breakdown. Going back to work
after three months off (including mindfulness training), she
committed to taking more care of herself. This included being
realistic about what she could manage, setting boundaries,

and deciding to spot and drop the perfectionist habits as they arose. As a result, she became more efficient, and actually got more work done than she had prior to her breakdown.

## Our own 'emotional soup'

When we are children, our developing brains and minds are like sponges. Where we are and who we're around shapes our brains, and particularly so when it comes to emotions and how we deal with them. The UK's reputation for the 'stiff upper lip' is one cultural example. At the other end of this scale is the Latin stereotype of overly expressed emotions. These are both variations of emotional reactions, habits that we were immersed in as we grew up and that may impact on how we respond to emotions and thoughts in our mindfulness practice. In both cases, a lack of balance can create difficulties.

The other influence is our family environment. We look to significant adults around us to understand how the world works and how to manage emotions. The ways in which these adults reacted to difficulties was coded into our developing brains. I call this the 'emotional soup' of the family. Reflecting on these experiences can tell us a lot about how we will likely relate to ourselves, our feelings and others in later life. Sometimes these habits can be so deep that it is only when we meet others who grew up in a different flavour of emotional soup that we even realize that things can be different.

Take a moment now to reflect on your own experience of emotions in your family. How were things when someone was sad, angry or fearful? It's possible you will have some version of this habitual response when you attempt to be non-reactive and non-judgemental with your emotions in your mindfulness practice. Mindfulness is an invitation to investigate old habits, see if they are still working for us and, if not, refine and retune them in a way that is more helpful for us right now, as adults.

Some people may not have had an adult model of gentleness, acceptance and curiosity about emotions when growing up. If this was the case for you, one tip is to think more widely in your life and notice people who do manage emotions and challenges skilfully. Observing role models can be very helpful. It taps into an innate learning mechanism – imitation. It is not that you want to copy them exactly, but you can 'fake it till you make it', using their behaviour as a guide.

### Do I need a mindfulness teacher?

Some individuals will definitely benefit from having a teacher in order to most safely commence their dive into the body and mind. Research confirms that having a teacher who has a good depth of personal experience will definitely have a positive impact on your training. Where you find this teacher depends on where you access mindfulness training (see more on this in Chapter 5).

The spiritual traditions provide guides of various levels of expertise, and you will also find peers who are more experienced who can share their knowledge with you. In the secular setting, you may find a teacher in the community, or via a health service or charity.

If you can't access a teacher for any reason, videos and web resources are plentiful. Always listen with a critical ear, assessing for yourself if what the person is saying is helpful. At a certain point, you will benefit from connecting with other mindfulness practitioners, as sharing experiences will accelerate your learning. But you can start right now, curating your own learning experience (see the box opposite).

**In summary**

In this chapter we've outlined some considerations that will make your mindfulness exploration more fruitful. Take time to consider both your external environment and internal (habits, personality, experiences). Finally, if you are someone who has a long history of relating to the present, your body, yourself or others in problematic ways, you may benefit from more support as you engage in this journey of self-development so don't be afraid to seek out help, perhaps from your doctor or a therapist. And remember: mindfulness isn't about a quick fix. To really change habits and feel calmer and more contented in the long-term, slow and steady wins the race.

## FOCUS ON CURATING YOUR OWN LEARNING EXPERIENCE

Ask yourself the following questions and use your responses to get you started on the mindfulness path. Focusing on this will make your attempts more personalized and therefore more efficient.

- How deep do you want to go? Do you need to pull up a few weeds or uproot a decades-old tree?
- What are you willing to commit to in terms of practice (frequency, duration, location)?
- How and when will you get started?
- Who might help or hinder you?
- How do you like to learn (reading, writing, watching, listening or moving)?
- How will you remember to be gentle with yourself?
- Did any personality traits described in this chapter resonate (and how will you take this into account)?

Keep a note of your answers. They will likely need updating as you start exploring. And what can you do right now to take a step in your desired direction? Perhaps download an app, search for a local class, or put some time in your diary to explore mindfulness.

# CHAPTER 5

What are the key ways
to develop mindfulness?

There are multiple routes to developing your innate mindfulness skills. In the previous chapter, suggestions were made to help you decide how you can best approach mindfulness training. In this chapter, we'll look at some key considerations that will help you find the best mindfulness training route for you. We'll also unpack three core exercises you can get going with right now. These exercises showcase how engaging mindfully in a few simple ways can have a profound impact. They are exercises that you'll encounter on any mindfulness training course, but they can also be done anywhere, anytime, and don't need special equipment. In addition, we'll take a look at the power of mindful communication, which is an incredible everyday mindfulness skill to cultivate.

## What are the various training considerations?

You may feel more than a little overwhelmed with choice when it comes to selecting the best approach to your mindfulness training. There's no right or wrong way to start; the most important thing is that you match the approach with your expectations. Don't expect a half-day workshop to totally transform your mind or an app to cure depression overnight. But do expect regular practice to gradually transform how you relate to any experience. Also, are you interested in self-transcendence or self-development? Your answer to this may lead you to access mindfulness in a spiritual or secular setting.

## Spiritual setting

Many spiritual traditions and faith practices from both the East (Buddhism, Taoism, Sufism) and West (Quaker, other Christian) offer routes to develop awareness that either overtly include mindfulness or have practices that tap into the same brain networks. They offer a life-long path to expand awareness in the service of connecting to the Divine. Spiritual or religious paths are usually well-defined, formalized and supported by a community. Finding a suitable spiritual teacher or guru is no small matter, however. Take your time and explore your options carefully before committing to a certain route.

## Self-development setting

If your intention is general self-development, secular training may be more suitable. You might find a MBSR or MBCT group advertised at your local health or community centre, or via a local charity. Some spiritual centres are also now offering secular mindfulness training programmes.

This training is typically a group of 12–20 individuals, meeting for 2–3 hours a week, to get basic instruction in mindfulness from an experienced (usually secular) mindfulness practitioner and teacher. You'll additionally be encouraged to practise by yourself for 45 minutes a day, so, to do this programme justice, I recommend ensuring you are able to make this time commitment before enrolling.

You may need or like to take a course tailored for a specific group, and these exist, too. For example, there are courses for children, young people, parents, creatives, corporate workers – you name it, there will likely be a mindfulness course based around it. More information on some specific courses can be found in the Further Reading section at the back of this book.

### Does your motivation match your intention?

Are you ready for formal training or just wanting to dip a toe in the water with informal practices? Remember, the same practices can be used for both routes (see the Try It box on page 108). If you have a modest intention to be more aware of the present and have time to relax in it, then a mindful colouring book or a nature-based activity is a relatively easy option to access. If your intention is to arrive at work less stressed and more focused, then informal and short practices may be sufficient. An app, workbook, an introductory workshop or a short course would give you the necessary tools to get started.

Although these quick approaches have their obvious benefits, without formal guidance, they can sometimes be more distraction than mindfulness training. For this reason, refer back to the 4-step 'mindful moment' cycle on page 46 while you engage in them to see if you are really developing your mindfulness potential.

If you have a high level of motivation and really want to fine-tune your attention, increase your productivity and develop your capacity to relate more deeply to others, a formal course like the MBSR or MBCT programmes (see page 80) would be a good starting point. These could be completed in a group or by following a programne in book form, such as MBCT-based *Finding Peace in a Frantic World* by Mark Williams and Danny Penman. If you like to work with practices that use your moving body, you could complete the Body In Mind training course in my book *Mindfulness in Motion*.

## What else do I need to think about?

Your personal learning preferences will also impact on your choice of approach. There are four things to consider:

**1** The frequency of your training (paced/intensive)
**2** The source of instruction you follow (self-guided/taught)
**3** How you will learn (group/individual/real-life/online)
**4** Your learning style (verbal/visual/auditory/kinaesthetic)

### Training frequency

Depending on your expectations, you might select a taught mindfulness course, which could be an intensive period of training spaced out over a couple of months. Alternatively, you might want to start with a drop-in group, allowing you to dip in when it suits you.

## TRYIT PRACTISING FORMALLY VERSUS INFORMALLY

Try a Mindfulness of the Posture exercise (see page 115) as both a formal and informal practice to learn the similarities and distinctions between the two. Whereas formal practices are deliberate times in the day when you stop to do just this activity, you should treat informal practices like mini breaks in the day – pauses for you to connect to the present moment.

**Formal:** Commit to one 3–5 minute formal posture exercise at a set time each day for at least ten days. Set an alarm on your phone or an appointment in your diary to help you remember.

**Informal:** Periodically focus attention on your posture. Become aware of the muscles, skin, and any places of relaxation or tension in the body. Where is there slumping or rigidity? Would it be more comfortable to put your posture into the alert–relaxed mode (see page 41)? How does this impact on your mental state? If you can, use the mindfulness bell app, a ring that goes off periodically throughout the day to remind you just to check 'Am I present?' Use it to prompt you to focus on your posture.

## Finding the right learning source

I highly recommend learning in a group. As well as providing a source of motivation and support from like-minded individuals, this environment allows you to hear about all the other minds in the room and gain a lot of extra learning from your peers. But this may not be for everyone. Some mindfulness teachers offer individual training options. They might run through mindfulness training books with you, guiding you through the exercises and ensuring you have grasped the key learning points and applications. Or you may find a personal coach or therapist who weaves mindfulness into their way of more generally supporting you.

## Guided or self-taught?

Guidance from an experienced teacher will enable you to recognize and deal with the personal blind spots that you might miss on your own. Independent practice will still be required, and apps and audios can help with this aspect. However, using an app alone will not be as effective as having a teacher to give you personalized feedback.

Research in the healthcare setting has shown that the level of mindfulness experience (rather than the professional discipline) of the teacher is of key importance. Ask your teacher about their personal experience of mindfulness and their training route. However, if you are approaching mindfulness with an existing health condition, check with a professional who knows about your condition whether standard mindfulness courses are ok for you, or seek out a teacher who specializes in your particular needs.

If you'd rather teach yourself, you can design your own programme, and find materials, such as workbooks, guided audios or online courses, to suit your learning style. This way, you can choose your own methods, pace and route. It's a great way to explore mindfulness but may have limitations if your intention is to truly transform, rather than just tame your mind.

### In real life or online?

If you can't physically get to a class or a teacher for any reason, then online training is a good option. Online groups have various ways to connect participants and a teacher, but you may miss the direct personal contact experienced in a group. Additionally, it may be difficult for the teacher to give more subtle guidance during the exercises. But this depends on your approach to the task.

If you are relatively healthy and engaging in mindfulness, the evidence suggests roughly equal benefits for online versus face-to-face training. The important thing to do is get going. Online options bring many advantages. Reminders, pings, email prompts can all help you to remember and prioritize practice. If you do decide that training online is for you, make sure you are only doing that activity and not just listening to the teacher while also cooking dinner!

**Your learning style**

Think about how you learn best. My preferred style is through the body. I'm considered a kinaesthetic learner. You might prefer to learn through verbal, visual or auditory routes. If you are not sure of your style, keep your options open and try a few different ways of learning to see what you prefer.

There are plenty of books out there for verbal learners. Auditory learners can access secular and spiritual talks and audio practices on the web. Visual learners are less well catered for (although see the 4-step diagram on page 46 as this is a strong visual learning aid); you may also find watching teachers delivering talks helpful. Kinaesthetic learners can augment formal mindfulness training with a tai chi or yoga class.

Having reviewed the key considerations as you select your training option, let's now unpack some common exercises. For three key exercises – Mindful Walking, Mindfulness of the Posture and Mindfulness of the Breath – you will learn:

- What makes the exercise mindful
- Top tips and common confusions

- Who the exercise might be best for
- Adaptations and advanced variations

## What is 'mindful walking'?

For most adults walking is an automatic activity we've been doing most of our lives. We once had to concentrate on it when learning as toddlers, but now we're mostly unaware of what we're doing when walking. *Mindful* walking brings this automatic process out into the light of our present moment, non-judgemental and non-reactive awareness. It's one of the richest mindfulness exercises and if you can nail this, you are well on your way to mindful living.

### It is mindful because ...

Movements that repeatedly co-occur are 'chunked' together by the brain. This time-saving device means we execute the 'walking' command automatically and can do many other tasks at the same time, such as checking our phones.

In mindful walking, we become interested in the sub-units of walking (including 'lift foot', 'swing leg', 'place foot' and 'shift weight') and how we transition between them. This allows us to see the smaller units that make up 'walking', and disrupts automatic programs in our brain. We are then better prepared to do the same with our mental habits, whether that is an unhealthy comparison cycle or an anxious planning loop.

Breaking these down into chunks is what breaks our mental habits and gives us a chance to build healthier ways of coping.

Walking provides a rich array of sensations arising from your hips, legs, knees, ankles and feet. You can choose to focus in on a single body part, such as the soles of the feet, or use a wider focus, taking in the whole body. By following the movement as it unfolds, your attention will be in the present moment, engaged with bodily sensations and how these change with movement. As usual, at some point your mind will wander, perhaps to thinking about walking, or to something else (such as planning an email or deciding what to eat later). Keeping in mind the 4-step 'mindful moment' cycle (see page 46), when you notice mind wandering, say to yourself, 'Oh, this is not walking' and gently but firmly refocus attention on walking.

### Top tips

Formal mindful walking is harder than it sounds! It is best done:

- At home, in a park or other quiet public space without too many distractions
- For 5–10 minutes initially (making walking your sole activity), then working up to longer durations (45 minutes)

Informal practice can turn any routine walk (across the lobby, down a corridor at home or work) into mindful walking.

## Best for

- Busy minds and busy lives (mums pushing prams can try this)
- Those who regularly commute
- Those who struggle with seated practices
- Those who usually do sitting practice (see how it is to be mindful when more of your brain is engaged by movement)
- Older adults (to increase the ability to sense information from the feet and ankles and reduce fear of falling)

## Common confusions

You don't *have* to move in slow motion when doing mindful walking, but it will make the practice more effective. Slowing down gives your brain much more detail about your body and mind, and will more thoroughly interrupt the automatic programming of the movement. The Focus On box on page 117 suggests how you might play with the speed of mindful actions such as walking as a deliberate exercise.

## Adaptations and advanced techniques

Challenge yourself to walk mindfully in busier environments, such as on a train or busy street. Map out some easier and some harder mindful walking routes just as you might select a hard or easy run on a fitness app. Practise attending to the intention to move as it arises, and before you actually move. Observe the decision to move, the body's preparation and the micro-moment of choice before each individual movement that emerges when we learn how to act with awareness. Try exploring the intentions behind each separate walking element (leg lift, swing, placement, etc).

## What is 'mindfulness of the posture'?

Paying full and focused attention to your posture at a given moment, whether you are sitting or standing, is mindfulness of the posture. We already looked at finding an alert–relaxed posture (see page 41), and have also used this exercise to explore formal and informal practice earlier in this chapter.

Keeping in mind the 4-step 'mindful moment' cycle (see page 46) will not only train your awareness, but also counteract any postural insults inflicted on your body over time with extended sitting and neck-bending.

### It is mindful because ...

As with all mindfulness exercises, when you focus your attention on the sensory information coming into your brain from your posture – your head, neck, shoulders, full length of your torso – your mind will wander. Don't worry, it's all part of the training. Choose your attentional focus – it could be narrow, wide, moving or still – and observe without trying to modify what's going on. When you become aware of your mind wandering, say to yourself, 'Oh, this is no longer posture' and gently but firmly refocus your attention as intended.

This exercise may prompt awareness of aches and pains, and awaken a desire for things to be different. Try to relate to your body in a gentle, non-reactive way, no matter what you encounter.

## Top tips

An optimal posture that is alert and relaxed is your aim. Alert your spine, pulling up as you breathe in and releasing wherever possible as you breathe out. Look out for:

- being either too alert and rigid (sergeant major)
- being too relaxed and slumped (surfer)
- how your posture changes over the day and in relation to specific thoughts and feelings that emerge

## Best for

- Desk-bound workers
- Those working on laptops and tablets at home, or in cafés that don't have ergonomic desk arrangements
- Anyone who carries multiple, heavy bags
- Anyone who regularly uses a smartphone (check how your neck feels)
- Anyone who spends a lot of time driving

One of my students who committed to this practice noticed a frequent pain in her left shoulder. It occurred to her that she carried a heavy handbag on this side. She made the way she carried her bag her mindfulness practice. Moving slowly, paying attention and staying curious, she broke the habit of putting her bag on her left shoulder. With mindfulness she

## FOCUS ON **MINDFULNESS AT DIFFERENT SPEEDS**

It's useful to try changing your pace during mindfulness practices that are based on movement, so you can notice how your brain commands your body in relation to speed. For example, the next time you try Mindful Walking, see if you can maintain the same level of attention when you walk faster or slower than your normal speed. Another good exercise is to mindfully answer your phone. Lots of us have strong emotional ties to our phones. Deliberately slow down the movement of your shoulder, arm and hand as you reach out, and observe any sensations related to the slow movement, as well as other sensations (thoughts, feelings or associations) in the periphery.

Where else in your life might a deliberate change of pace in either direction (slower/faster) allow you to see things that were not previously in your awareness?

could check her actions against her bigger intention to be kinder to her body, and from this, choose the best course of action.

## Common confusions

Mindfulness of the posture can often drift into mindfulness of the breath in the body. If this happens, check if you *chose* to switch objects or if your attention was *automatically* drawn to the rhythmic movement of the breath. Some people choose to visualize a string pulling the head and spine up to help with posture awareness. While this technique supports a healthy posture, creating visual imagery can pull you away from directly sensing the present moment via bodily sensations, so be careful you don't get lost in this imagery.

## Adaptations and advanced techniques

If you plan to do extended practices (for longer than 40 minutes duration), it will help to work out a posture that is as comfortable as possible, without being so comfortable that you fall asleep. A variety of cross-legged, lying down or kneeling positions are available to you. Just see what works for your body and level of flexibility through trial and error. Try to make your habitual posture one of alert relaxation, no matter what you are doing, and become aware of your posture during everyday activities such as showering, washing up or waiting for the bus.

## What is 'mindfulness of the breath'?

As described in Chapter 2, mindfulness of the breath is a key practice. It's not a 'breathing exercise', as there is no attempt to control or change the breath. Simply, make the breath the focus of your attention.

## This is mindful because ....

When focusing on the breath, you are attending to the subtle sensations experienced with each breath, sensory information that can only be in the here and now; not in the past or the future. You may experience these sensations at your nostril area or moving through your body. However it occurs for you, when your mind wanders, just follow the 4-step 'mindful moment' cycle and say to yourself, 'Oh, this is not breath', then gently but firmly refocus your attention on the breath.

## Top tips

Try the following variations on mindfulness of the breath:

- First sense the breath as it moves through the body. Then move your attention to explore changes near the nostrils.
- Do not be alarmed by common task-related mind-wandering, including thoughts such as 'Am I breathing?' or 'How am I breathing?' or 'How long or short is my breath?' Over-thinking the breath can lead to changes in the breath, which reinforce the thoughts that there is something

wrong with it. Note this as 'task-related mind-wandering' and trust that you do know how to breathe!

- If helpful, count a few breaths to help you settle into the practice, then remember to drop the counting.

## Best for

- Transitioning between activities, whatever these may be. Try three mindful breaths in these moments. Use the first breath to acknowledge where you have just come from; the second to ground you in the body and the here and now; the third to set your intention for the next activity.
- Soothing agitated minds. Even if you lose the focus on the breath and have to come back once, twice, 50 or even 100 times, that's ok. Keep trying. Eventually, if you stay with the breath, your mind will settle.
- Preparing for difficult conversations or experiences. Observing your breath will give you a sense of your emotional landscape. With practice, you'll learn that attending to your breath will help you to carry out any task more efficiently.

## Common confusions

If you become aware that you're trying to control or change the breath at all, you have moved into a breathing exercise and are no longer using the breath as the object for focused attention training. Just watch, don't add anything to the task.

Also be careful not to start analysing the breath, particularly if you find it is short or shallow. It may be altered if you are feeling a strong emotion. Stay with it in an accepting, non-reactive way and, in most cases, it will settle of its own accord. Some people count the total number of breaths or use counting to determine the length of the breath. This is useful if done mindfully and with clear intention. However, don't get attached to counting. Try without counting at some point and notice how the experience is different.

## Adaptations and advanced techniques

Despite what I've just said above, you can use breath-counting as a way to deliberately understand more about your mind. Counting can easily become automatic – just see what happens if you set yourself the surprisingly hard task of counting 300 breaths. This exercise reveals a lot about the naturally high levels of distraction in most minds. Enter with low expectations of success and a bit of light humour! You can also explore the natural suspension of breath that occurs between the in and out breath, when breathing has settled and/or you are doing longer practices. Spiritual traditions have a wealth of detailed practices exploring this moment (considered by some as a bridge representing the transition between life and death). For now, however, don't get too agitated or excited by anything you experience, just observe and watch how your mind plays in this area.

## How can I communicate mindfully?

One practice that will make a huge difference to your life is mindful communication. You can start in the very next conversation you have and make both the listening and speaking parts your mindfulness practice. Simply set your intention to fully attend to what the other person is saying, no matter what. Notice if you are pulled away from listening, by task-related mind-wandering, for example, or because you are lost in memories, associations or mental activity triggered by the person's words. Or you might be drawn into a positive or negative emotional reaction to what they are saying, or in planning your response. Develop your non-reactive and non-judgemental awareness, choosing to calmly return your full attention to their words. Not only will you gather and retain more information about what has been said, your brain will also process more non-verbal cues from the speaker's body and you'll become more sensitive to what is *not* being said.

When it's your turn to speak, pause for a moment to give yourself time to match the intentions behind your words with the words themselves. Consider this: is it more important to preserve your relationship, be right or get a certain outcome? Or do you have a broader intention, for example, to communicate wisely and with courage? When you then speak, your words will hopefully feel calm, compassionate and in alignment with your underlying intentions.

Giving someone this deep quality of attention when they are speaking has real impact for both parties – it feels like quite a different interaction altogether. We are so used to receiving and giving relatively poor attention in our modern world that the novelty of this level of attentional focus can generate both positive and negative reactions! As with any skill, it takes practice and gets better the more you do it, so try it as often as you can.

## In summary

In this chapter we've looked at a variety of routes to develop your mindfulness. There are also many other activities you are doing all the time, whether eating, doing the dishes, folding laundry or mowing the lawn, which can be done mindfully. If you have an understanding of what it means to be mindful, any activity is a chance to practice. Read on to find out what life could be like if we were all in these contented, non-reactive, present-moment states more of the time. What would the world be like if everyone paid a bit more kindly attention in an ongoing manner?

# CHAPTER 6
What are the future possibilities with mindfulness?

From reading this far, you've learned about both the simplicity and complexity that is mindfulness. You have discovered that mindfulness is a type of awareness, and one we can access at any time if we apply a little concentration. You've learned methods to train and enhance this awareness to give it the three important characteristics that turn ordinary awareness into mindfulness: first, focusing solely on the present moment; second, being non-reactive, and third, being non-judgemental. And you've seen why the simple suggestion to 'be mindful' is often quite hard. Having taken all of this in, try using the Focus On box (opposite) to consider where in your life *now* you would benefit most from mindfulness.

## How can I take my personal journey forward?

With the tools provided in this book you are well placed to make a good start on your personal journey with mindfulness. Remember, there is no right way. Only the way that is most helpful for you at this moment. Hold these three concepts in mind to help you progress: act with awareness, embrace life's challenges and find your own way.

### Act with awareness

In choosing mindfulness exercises, or making any decisions, commit to acting with awareness. This simply means knowing what you are doing as you are doing it and, ideally, just

## FOCUS ON IDENTIFYING HOW MINDFULNESS CAN MOST BENEFIT YOU

Living mindfully can change all spheres of our life, but is best approached in a deliberate and targeted way. As such, it's extremely valuable to take some time out to consider in which areas of your life mindfulness could most help you. This may be relationships, career, leisure, purpose, finance, health or anything else.

1 Where in your life do you find yourself overly distracted? Where would it help to have more focus?

2 Where in your life are you particularly reactive or overly emotional? Where would it help to be calmer and more considered?

3 In what areas of your life are you overly hard on yourself or others? Where might you resolve a problem more quickly if you approached it gently?

4 Where would it be helpful to approach things in a more curious, calm and kind manner? How would you use the time and energy released if you did this?

before. Aware of the urge to speak or move, your mindfulness training will help you check in with the underlying 'why' of your words/actions. This, in turn, will allow you to determine if your broader intentions are going to be met. Ask yourself, 'Is this action in line with how I intend to be in the world?' This requires you to know and set your intentions, use these to guide your subsequent actions, and respond calmly rather than react negatively when you see you're going off track.

### Embrace life's challenges

Life throws challenges at us all. Events such as unexpected illness or sudden changes in circumstance often force us to revisit what's important and may require dramatic modification of our intentions. Luckily, intentions are flexible. There are also natural points where conditions change and it is helpful to review our intentions. For example, when we move into or out of relationships or work, become parents, or as we age. Could you navigate the next transition in *your* life with more awareness of intentions? This would ensure you were being true to yourself in the moment, not a version of yourself from the past or an imagined future self.

A mindful response to a crisis asks us to dig deep and discover who we really are. It means taking full advantage of any learning opportunities, and not wasting energy wishing things were different and struggling against the experience.

**Find your own way**

As explored already, you can choose either formal or informal ways to develop mindfulness. The important thing, no matter which approach you decide on, is to follow the 4-step 'mindful moment' cycle on page 46 to ensure that it is done in an informed and efficient way.

For one person, mindful living may be a commitment to being more present in everyday activities, such as walking in nature, and engaging in a creative endeavour. For another, it may be a decision to use moments of challenge as your non-reactivity training, such as working mindfully with road rage or a difficult neighbour. Deciding to approach these daily frustrations mindfully, rather than reacting explosively to them, provides vital training that will support you when bigger challenges arise.

Another person might experiment with how it feels to live with more kindness and compassion as their over-arching intention. Just going into a meeting with a difficult colleague with the intention to 'be open' held in mind can make a huge difference. It gets easier the more you practice.

You may be ready for (or need) a more dedicated route, committing to a course or a longer training. This level of intention-setting will help to ensure your efforts pay off.

## What can I expect if I keep practising?

With continued practice of mindfulness you will slowly but surely start to experience life differently – being more present, less reactive and more compassionate to both yourself and others. Expect that things will change – sometimes dramatically, and sometimes slowly and subtly. Expect to be surprised, excited, challenged, bemused, confused and sometimes uncertain about what is going on. When these things are happening you really know you're on the right track and learning.

### Being more present

At first, you'll likely be shocked at discovering how distracted you have been. As you reduce distractions and increase your capacity to be present, the richness of the life right in front of you is likely to evolve and become all the more apparent.

Being present will not only allow you to take better care of yourself, but will also enhance your relationships. You'll see people as they are now and not how they were ten years ago or even yesterday. Imagine someone you've had a long-standing disagreement with. What would it be like to see them tomorrow and engage with them as if meeting for the first time? Think of the possibilities and opportunities that open up when we are not wedded to our expectations of how things are (or afraid that they may not be as we want them).

## Being less reactive

Increased awareness can reveal aspects of yourself that are challenging. Mindfulness allows us to be non-reactive precisely at this moment. With this stance, we can respond more calmly. Even when it seems things are really not ok, we see that we can cope. Rather than seeing illness, ageing and death as personal attacks, for example, we come to understand that this is the lot of all humans. The Focus On box on page 134 provides some reflective questions to help you understand how your relationship with yourself can change through ongoing mindfulness.

## Being more compassionate

During the mindfulness of the breath exercise on pages 50–51, when you noticed things like, 'Oh, thoughts about dinner tonight, that's not breath!' and applied a more gentle tone of voice with yourself, you probably got back to your task fairly fast. Discovering that being less harsh on yourself speeds your learning is a key stage in mindfulness development. Repeated practice with 'small' moments of self-compassion like this trains you to be able to apply the same orientation of mind in your wider life.

Relationships are one place where we can really see benefits here. Relating more kindly to ourselves, particularly our emotions, automatically helps us to relate more kindly to others. Understanding that we react when we are in pain or upset, makes it easier to understand when others react. If you've been too gentle (with others) at the expense of yourself, the self-compassion training of mindfulness will help you set appropriate boundaries with others. This is the firm side of compassion. Equally, those who have been too firm with themselves or others learn how to cut themselves some slack and know that its ok not to be perfect/first/right all the time.

Do take care, however, that your desire to develop yourself doesn't turn into striving for perfection. Also, don't be alarmed by the extent of judging and reactivity you uncover; it's important to try not to judge or react when you see it!

## What happens with continued mindfulness practice?

Gradually, and over time, mindful states become more frequent and stable, and the mind becomes naturally more inclined toward compassion, both to self and others. Let's look at highly developed mindfulness skills in both secular and spiritual settings, and see where these might overlap.

### Secular

In today's world, we have a new generation of secular mindfulness practitioners. These may be people who have met mindfulness at work, school or online. They may or may not be interested in deeper spiritual questions, but are certainly interested in the benefits of mindfulness for body and mind. They have a variety of intentions and various levels of commitment to practice. But how they are learning and training is very different to how mindfulness has traditionally been taught in spiritual and philosophical settings.

And yet, slowly and surely, more and more people are using this method to wake up from living life on autopilot. They are learning how to consciously check in with what's really important to them rather than waiting until unexpected events force them to do so. They are learning that they do have choices, and the power of setting intentions. Mindfulness practitioners often make choices that go against the grain of society's habits to acquire more, work more, amass wealth. Mindfulness teaches us to live with what we need, rather than what we want.

**Spiritual**

Monks and nuns from various monastic and contemplative traditions have made living mindfully their vocation. With decades of precise, formalized training and few distractions, it's interesting to consider how they see the world. As one mountain-dwelling Tibetan yogi once let slip, 'Although I do appear like a human person outwardly, my mental state is so different.' Their whole experience of reality and awareness changes from that of the everyday person.

## FOCUS ON USING MINDFULNESS WHEN THINGS GO WRONG

We often create more problems when things go wrong by reacting in overly dramatic or pessimistic ways. This prevents us from seeing that, even within the suffering, there may be some learning that can help us. Notice what happens in your body as you reflect on the questions below. Be alert to any ways your mind tries to move you away from even thinking about them.

How do you relate to your own personal difficulties, frustrations, illness or rejection? And how do you relate to the problems of those close to you? How do you relate to the pain of those outside your immediate environment, for example refugees or those living in war-torn states, or to the huge problems facing our planet, from climate change to social inequality?

Mindfulness doesn't magically make bad and sad things disappear. But, if we can remain mindful and curious even when things are not ok, creative solutions can often be found. Being less reactive means what's already happening is not compounded by knee-jerk reactions that make things worse.

Their expanded awareness means they can lead life following the more powerful sensations of the heart. A heart-centred life de-emphasizes the conceptual, intellectual way of relating to self and the world and promotes living with the intention to provide a model of unconditional love. This compassionate stance is not a soft option – it takes training and courage.

## Where spiritual and secular meet

Secular and spiritual mindfulness are separate entities, yet they remain entwined. Many of the secular programmes have been developed by lay spiritual practitioners. So, can they really be fully secular, and does it matter if everyone brings their own intention to the practice anyway?

It is almost inevitable that secular practitioners, with continued practice, will start to ask questions about their experience that take them off the knowledge maps of Western science and into the spiritual domain. Focused attention training when applied to awareness itself starts to open up a different space of enquiry, and one that is currently best defined by the spiritual traditions. In general, it seems that there is increasing mainstream interest in more spiritual questions, and mindfulness may be a bridge for many to start engaging in these deeper questions, such as 'What is my purpose on this planet?' or 'How can I best contribute to the world?'

## Where is there innovation in the mindfulness field?

The blending of Eastern and Western traditions, the addition of modern science, and the application of 21st-century methods of teaching, all make this a very exciting time for mindfulness. With the secular door to mindfulness now wide open, there has been an explosion of adaptations and innovations as mindfulness enters different settings as varied as healthcare, education, the workplace and beyond. The application of mindfulness is being re-shaped and re-modelled as it enters more and more spheres of life. Here are a few examples of what might be on the horizon.

### Innovations from neuroscience

In this book, my main intention is to share the 4-step cycle on page 46, to give you an understanding of the neural networks that need to be 'worked out' for you to gain the benefits of mindfulness and build your own unique approach to living mindfully. This innovative use of neuroscience data as applied to learning and exploring mindfulness will help you see that any activity really can be done mindfully, even cutting the lawn, tying shoelaces, preparing and eating dinner. Check, did you set your intention? Check, did you choose to focus your attention on just that one thing you were doing? Did you calmly, compassionately note when your mind wandered and then commit to refocus? If so, you have been developing your mindfulness and working out your brain.

## Innovations in how mindfulness is being applied

On the back of scientific evidence, mindfulness is now being introduced to settings far beyond healthcare (which is where it first appeared in a secular setting). Bringing mindfulness into schools, offices and elsewhere has required adaptations to ensure the methods are suitable for the intention of the work in these contexts. Often this has involved 'traditional' exercises with a modern twist, taking the best of all worlds to maximize learning. There are some quite mind-boggling possibilities with all of this. What if all offices were full of more mindful workers? What if all schools were full of mindful kids and teachers? What kind of adults might these children become? And how might decisions made by global leaders be different if they were mindful?

## 'Whole systems' mindfulness

One innovation is in attempts to create whole systems modelled on mindfulness. The Dragon Café in London is an example of this. It is a creative healing space for the community to explore issues around mental health, fully infused with mindfulness. The team there use mindful processes in their decision-making, and team members and volunteers at the café are trained personally in mindfulness, which impacts on all interactions. Mindfulness is also offered (in a creative format) to those who visit the café. This is a space where vulnerability and 'dis-ease' are given non-reactive and non-judgemental treatment. It is a living model of how to be aware of even the most painful and difficult experiences in a mindful way to promote growth. Compassion is there, but so is intent, all underpinned by two key questions: How do you want to make sense of this experience? And what do you need right now?

Critically, the café is about connection and the recognition that while the reasons for our individual distress may be unique, any feelings of, loss, fear, anger, abandonment, happiness and joy are common to us all. The success of the Dragon Café is attracting widespread attention from service providers and healthcare workers. Can you imagine if our public healthcare systems or big businesses were operating like this? It's not an easy option, it takes courage and commitment, but the Dragon Café shows us it is possible.

### In summary

Mindfulness continues to evolve. It was ever thus. The more we peel back and return to our innate mindful capacity, the greater the chance we have to live together harmoniously on this planet. Our human condition connects us all, including the pain, the shame, the joys and the tears. Being open and unafraid of our vulnerabilities helps us better connect, learn and grow. Mindfulness is the vehicle to help us traverse these parts of ourselves so that we can all thrive.

# What next?

The notion of a world full of more mindful citizens, including the next generation of leaders and influencers, is a great source of hope and one that is not beyond the impossible.

We might then be able to see the real cost of 'modern development' and recognize the organizational and cultural habits that are leading us down unhelpful paths. Mindfulness would give us the courage to stand up and say, 'Hey, wait a minute, is this really what we intended?' It may be hard to take a mindful look at some of the things we've done to each other and the planet. But with the curiosity to really see what's going on, the courage to do something different, and compassion at the heart of all decisions, we could undo old habits and create systems and communities that nurture rather than deplete us.

More mindful citizens would not get caught up in judgement or hold on so tightly to old ideas. They would see these for what they are – habits or thoughts that once served a purpose, but that are no longer useful. That's all. Time to let go and change.

So now, here, in this moment ... what are we choosing? How do we want to orient our collective mind? If you were to wipe the slate clean and start again, what sort of world do you want to live in? Doesn't a more mindful one seem appealing?

# Further reading

Adams, J (2016) *Mindfulness Leadership for Dummies*

Chambers, R. & Ulbrick, M (2016) *Mindful relationships: creating genuine connection with ourselves and others*

Fox, K. C., Nijeboer, S., Dixon, M. L., Floman, J. L., Ellamil, M., Rumak, S. P., . . . Christoff, K. (2014). 'Is meditation associated with altered brain structure? A systematic review and meta-analysis of morphometric neuroimaging in meditation practitioners.' *Neuroscience and Biobehavioral Reviews*, 43, 48-73.

Hasenkamp, W, Wilson-Mendenhall, CD., Duncan, E. & Barsalou, W. (2012) 'Mind wandering and attention during focused meditation: A fine-grained temporal analysis of fluctuating cognitive states.' *NeuroImage* 59, 750–760.

Hölzel, B. K., Lazar, S. W., Gard, T., Schuman-Olivier, Z., Vago, D. R., & Ott, U. (2011). 'How does mindfulness meditation work? Proposing mechanisms of action from a conceptual and neural perspective.' *Perspectives on Psychological Science*, 6(6), 537-559.

Kabat-Zinn, J (2013) *Full Catastrophe Living (Revised Edition): Using the Wisdom of Your Body and Mind to Face Stress, Pain, and Illness*

Kabat-Zinn, M & Kabat-Zinn, J (1998) *Everyday Blessings: The inner work of mindful parenting*

Malinowski, P. (2013). 'Neural mechanisms of attentional control in mindfulness meditation.' *Frontiers in Neuroscience*, 7, 8.

Marturano, J (2015) *Finding the space to lead: a practical guide to mindful leadership*

Puddicombe, A (2013) *The Headspace Guide to... Mindful Eating: 10 Days to Finding Your Ideal Weight*

Russell, T (2015) *Mindfulness in Motion*

Shapiro, S. & White, C. (2014) *Mindful Discipline: A Loving Approach to Setting Limits and Raising an Emotionally Intelligent Child*

Tang, Y. Y., Hölzel, B. K., & Posner, M. I. (2015). 'The neuroscience of mindfulness meditation.' *Nature Reviews Neuroscience*, 16(4), 213-225.

Thich Nhat Hanh & Cheung, L (2011) *Savor: Mindful Eating, Mindful Life*

Wallace, A & Goleman, D (2006) *The Attention Revolution: Unlocking the Power of the Focused Mind*

Williams, M and Penman, D (2012) *Finding Peace in a Frantic world*

Vago, D. R., & Silbersweig, S. A. (2012). 'Self-Awareness, self-regulation, and self-transcendence (S-ART): A framework for understanding the neurobiological mechanisms of mindfulness.' *Frontiers in Human Neuroscience*, 6, 296.

Zeidan, F., Grant, J. A., Brown, C. A., McHaffie, J. G., & Coghill, R. C. (2012). 'Mindfulness meditation-related pain relief: Evidence for unique brain mechanisms in the regulation of pain.' *Neuroscience Letters*, 520(2), 165-173.

# Acknowledgments

There are too many students, teachers, guides, clients and supporters to mention. Interactions with each and every one have informed what is written in these pages. You have all given gifts of immeasurable value. Those friends and family who bore the brunt of this particular writing process, you know who you are and I thank you from the bottom of my heart for your patience, gentleness and (when needed) firmness!

Special thanks to Jo Childs my co-editor and mindfulness consultant for her patient help and support in the initial thinking and content shaping of this book. Also to Kelly Thompson and the team at Watkins, especially the amazing editorial support from Becky Miles whose gentle but firm guidance kept things on track.

# ABOUT THE AUTHOR

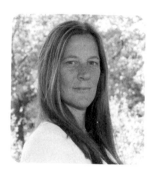

**DR TAMARA RUSSELL**

Dr Tamara Russell is an experienced clinical psychologist, martial artist and neuroscientist who brings a unique, multiple perspective to mindfulness teaching, thinking, therapy and research. Currently the Director of the Mindfulness Centre of Excellence in London and a visiting Lecturer at King's College London, she is also a mindfulness consultant, trainer and speaker in a wide variety of settings, including education and health. Tamara's first book by Watkins, *Mindfulness in Motion*, has been sold internationally.

# ABOUT THE SERIES

We hope you've enjoyed reading this book.
If you'd like to find out more about other therapies, practices
and phenomena that you've heard of and been curious about,
then do take a look at the other titles in our thought-provoking
**#WHATIS** series by visiting www.whatisseries.com

# #WHATIS

The growing list of dynamic books in this series will allow
you to explore a wide range of life-enhancing topics – sharing
the history, wisdom and science of each subject, as well as
its far-reaching practical applications and benefits. With each guide
written by a practising expert in the field, this new series challenges
preconceptions, demystifies the subjects in hand and encourages
you to find new ways to lead a more fulfilled, meaningful and
contented life.

## OTHER TITLES IN THE **#WHATIS** SERIES:

*What is a Near-Death Experience?* by Dr Penny Sartori
*What is Sound Healing?* by Lyz Cooper
*What is Hypnosis?* by Tom Fortes Mayer
*What is Numerology?* by Sonia Ducie
*What is Post-Traumatic Growth?* by Miriam Akhtar

# WATKINS

Sharing Wisdom Since
1893

The story of Watkins dates back to 1893, when the scholar of esotericism John Watkins founded a bookshop, inspired by the lament of his friend and teacher Madame Blavatsky that there was nowhere in London to buy books on mysticism, occultism or metaphysics. That moment marked the birth of Watkins, soon to become the home of many of the leading lights of spiritual literature, including Carl Jung, Rudolf Steiner, Alice Bailey and Chögyam Trungpa.

Today, the passion at Watkins Publishing for vigorous questioning is still resolute. Our wide-ranging and stimulating list reflects the development of spiritual thinking and new science over the past 120 years. We remain at the cutting edge, committed to publishing books that change lives.

## DISCOVER MORE . . .

Read our blog

Watch and listen to
our authors in action

Sign up to
our mailing list

## JOIN IN THE CONVERSATION

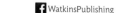 WatkinsPublishing  @watkinswisdom

 watkinsbooks  watkinswisdom 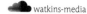 watkins-media

Our books celebrate conscious, passionate, wise and happy living.
Be part of the community by visiting

www.watkinspublishing.com